Psychiatric Aspects of Abortion

ISSUES IN
PSYCHIATRY

Joseph D. Bloom, M.D.
Series Editor

Psychiatric Aspects of Abortion

Edited by

Nada L. Stotland, M.D.

Director of Psychiatric Education,
Associate Professor of Clinical Psychiatry and Obstetrics and Gynecology,
The University of Chicago, Chicago, Illinois

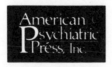

Washington, DC
London, England

Note: The authors have worked to ensure that all information in this book concerning drug dosages, schedules, and routes of administration is accurate as of the time of publication and consistent with standards set by the U.S. Food and Drug Administration and the general medical community. As medical research and practice advance, however, therapeutic standards may change. For this reason and because human and mechanical errors sometimes occur, we recommend that readers follow the advice of a physician who is directly involved in their care or the care of a member of their family.

Books published by the American Psychiatric Press, Inc., represent the views and opinions of the individual authors and do not necessarily represent the policies and opinions of the Press or the American Psychiatric Association.

Copyright © 1991 American Psychiatric Press, Inc.
ALL RIGHTS RESERVED
Manufactured in the United States of America on acid-free paper.
94 93 92 91 4 3 2 1
First Edition

American Psychiatric Press, Inc.
1400 K Street, N.W., Washington, DC 20005

Library of Congress Cataloging-in-Publication Data

Psychiatric aspects of abortion / edited by Nada L. Stotland.—1st ed.
    p.   cm.—(Issues in psychiatry)
   Includes bibliographical references and index.
   ISBN 0-88048-451-9 (alk. paper)
   1. Abortion—Psychological aspects.   2. Psychology, Pathological.
3. Psychotherapy.   4. Abortion—Social aspects.   I. Stotland, Nada Logan.
II. Series.
   [DNLM: 1. Abortion, Induced—psychology.   HQ 767 P974]
RG734.P79   1991
616.8'8'019—dc20
DNLM/DLC
for Library of Congress   90-14489
                                                                              CIP

British Library Cataloguing in Publication Data

A CIP record is available from the British Library.

To my mother,
Cyrel Dulsky Logan,
and
her mother,
Goldie Midlin,
who understood the importance of
choices about motherhood.

Contents

Contributors

Eileen Anderson, R.N., B.Sc.N., M.Ed.
Director of Nursing, Chilliwack General Hospital, Chilliwack, British Columbia, Canada

Irma J. Bland, M.D.
Associate Chair, Director of Clinical Services, Department of Psychiatry, LSU Medical Center, New Orleans, Louisiana

Susan J. Blumenthal, M.D., M.P.A.
Chief, Behavioral Medicine Program, National Institute of Mental Health, Rockville, Maryland; Clinical Associate Professor of Psychiatry, Georgetown University School of Medicine, Washington, DC

Carl Elliott, M.D.
Fellow, Center for Clinical Medical Ethics, University of Chicago Hospital, Chicago, Illinois

Judith H. Gold, M.D., F.R.C.P.(C)
Private practice; formerly Associate Professor, Department of Psychiatry, Dalhousi University, Halifax, Nova Scotia, Canada

Elisabeth K. Herz, M.D.
Director of Psychosomatic Obstetrical/Gynecological Program and Associate Professor, Department of Obstetrics/Gynecology and Psychiatry, George Washington University Medical Center, Washington, DC

John D. Lantos, M.D.
Assistant Professor of Pediatrics and Associate Director of the Center for Clinical Medical Ethics, University of Chicago Hospitals; Chief of Medical Staff, La Rabida Children's Hospital, Chicago, Illinois

Christine L. McHenry, M.D.
Fellow, Center for Clinical Medical Ethics, University of Chicago Hospitals, Chicago, Illinois

Sarah L. Minden, M.D.
Associate Physician, Division of Psychiatry, Brigham and Women's Hospital, Boston; Instructor in Psychiatry, Harvard Medical School; Senior Scientist, Law and Public Policy area, Abt Associates Inc., Cambridge, Massachusetts

Shaila Misri, M.D., F.R.C.P.(C)
Head of Consultation/Liaison Services, Department of Obstetrics and Gynecology, Grace Hospital; Head of PMS Clinic, University Hospital, Shaughnessy Site; Associate Clinical Professor, Departments of Psychiatry and Obstetrics/Gynecology, University of British Columbia, Vancouver, British Columbia, Canada

Lucile F. Newman, Ph.D.
Professor, Department of Community Health and Anthropology, Brown University, Providence, Rhode Island

Malkah T. Notman, M.D.
Clinical Professor of Psychiatry, Director of Academic Affairs, Harvard Medical School, Cambridge, Massachusetts

Miriam B. Rosenthal, M.D.
Director, Division of Behavioral Obstetrics and Gynecology and Consultation-Liaison Psychiatrist, MacDonald Hospital for Women and University Hospitals of Cleveland; Associate Professor of Reproductive Biology and Psychiatry, Case Western Reserve University School of Medicine, Cleveland, Ohio

Arden Rothstein, Ph.D.
Clinical Psychologist in private practice, New York City; Advanced Candidate in Psychoanalytic Training, The Psychoanalytic Institute, New York University Medical Center; at the time of the research reported, Assistant Professor of Psychiatry, Albert Einstein College of Medicine; also formerly Chief of Child and Adolescent Psychiatry, New York Hospital–Westchester Division and Assistant Professor of Psychology in Psychiatry, Cornell University Medical Center, New York, New York

Lynn T. Shepler, M.D.
Department of Psychiatry, Yale University School of Medicine, New Haven, Connecticut

Elisabeth C. Small, M.D.
Professor of Psychiatry and Clinical Associate Professor of Obstetrics and Gynecology, University of Nevada School of Medicine; Chief of Psychiatry, Veterans Administration Medical Center, Reno, Nevada

Nada L. Stotland, M.D.
Director of Psychiatric Education, Associate Professor of Clinical Psychiatry and Obstetrics and Gynecology, The University of Chicago, Chicago, Illinois

Florence R. Young, R.N., M.S.N.
Associate Clinical Professor, Frances Payne Bolton School of Nursing, Case Western Reserve University; Director of Nursing, MacDonald Hospital for Women, University Hospital of Cleveland, Cleveland, Ohio

Chapter 1

Psychiatric Issues in Abortion, and the Implications of Recent Legal Changes for Psychiatric Practice

Nada L. Stotland, M.D.

Psychiatry and Abortion: Recent History, Current Change

Inherent philosophical tensions, recent social controversy, and change in the judicial and legislative climate of the United States with regard to induced abortion raise questions for psychiatrists as citizens, as educators, and as specialized medical and mental health practitioners. This book was conceived in the spirit of reflection on the impact of the *Roe v. Wade* (1973) decision of the U.S. Supreme Court, which acknowledged the right of a woman to make decisions about the termination of early pregnancies in consultation with her health care provider and significant others. The book was developed in the context of a major change in the membership and rulings of the Supreme Court on the subject of abortion. It was to be a resource for the psychiatric practitioner, consolidating the results of an era of openness in reproductive decision making and considering the many facets of the subject: gender, race, ethnicity, age, history, values, ethics, law, and stage of gestation. Now it may also serve as a handbook for the psychiatrist grappling with the effects of recent political developments, judicial changes, and legislative controversies on the psychiatric health of individuals as patients and as members of our society and on the practice of psychiatry. Readers will note some overlap among chapters in terms of literature review and other issues; this overlap exists so that each chapter can be read and used on its own for clinical work, teaching, and consultation.

In the United States, in the years before the 1973 Supreme Court *Roe v. Wade* decision, which disallowed restrictions on early abortions, and in other countries with restricted access to medical abortion services, psychiatrists were often asked to serve on committees controlling access to abortion (Ford et al. 1971a). Many other psychiatrists confronted the situation in the office evaluations of individual patients (Bolter 1962). When a woman had to demonstrate that her life was at risk to justify an abortion, psychiatrists were called on to attest that a woman would commit suicide if her fetus were not aborted. An evaluation performed under these circumstances was skewed and limited. The woman, who would not have been a "patient" were it not for the law, was in the psychiatrist's office not to seek help for a psychiatric problem, but to accomplish a specific purpose (Ford et al. 1971b). She was constrained to reveal or describe only signs and symptoms she believed would help her achieve that end. The psychiatrist had to decide whether to try to deduce her "real" condition and whether and how to serve as a gatekeeper for the abortion procedure. Producing a report calculated to have the effect the woman desired was a distortion of the psychiatric diagnosis and treatment process (Bolter 1962). Refusing to cooperate consigned the woman to an unknown fate—possibly directly self-damaging behavior but, more likely, another psychiatric evaluation by a more sympathetic clinician, unwanted childbearing, or an illegal abortion posing significant risk of morbidity and mortality.

Residents in psychiatry were among those involved in such clinical situations. There is no record of educational techniques or guidelines used to help them organize their thinking, deal with cognitive and ethical questions, and handle their own values and feelings. How could psychiatric educators have developed an educational response to a situation in which the use of psychiatry was a political by-product but also one in which the practitioner might believe that cooperation was in the interest of the patient's mental health? The result was that trainees were often forced to handle these demanding and paradoxical problems without faculty support. Many of today's psychiatrists were trained under these circumstances. Now, as today's teachers and supervisors, we will face that dilemma again, at least in some states and circumstances.

The psychiatric literature in the pre-*Roe* era tended to focus on and question adverse psychological consequences of induced abortion (Pasnau 1972; Senay 1970). In the years after the *Roe v. Wade* decision, studies of abortion have asked richer questions and revealed more complex findings. The only women found to be at significant risk of psychiatric illness after abortions were those with histories of major psychiatric illness, those with serious psychosocial problems, and those whose decision to terminate a pregnancy was made under duress (Ewing and Rouse 1973). Sequelae, such as psychosis, are significantly more frequent after term delivery (David et al. 1981). The immediate precipitant of psychiatric complications is the problem of pregnancy (Ashton 1980). The circumstances that lead to pregnancy and the stress it imposes are at least as likely to play an etiological role in postabortion psychiatric illness as the abortion procedure. When doctors and patients work together without governmental constraint, they can use the psychotherapeutic process to explore the meanings and consequences of all courses of action in response to a possibly unwelcome pregnancy (Friedman et al. 1974).

The legal and social contexts of abortion and the expectations of doctors and patients have had a marked effect on (or even determined) abortion outcome. Few original studies have been published in the last 5 or 8 years. Perhaps the relevant questions had been answered. But it is more likely that growing pressure from groups adamantly opposed to induced abortion, which closed many clinics, also decreased research funding for psychiatric aspects of abortion and made scientists and clinicians wary of working on the subject. The immediate past U.S. surgeon general, C. Everett Koop, seemed to have been chosen for his post on the basis of his antiabortion history. He was ordered by President Ronald Reagan to write a report on the medical and psychological effects of abortion. The American Psychiatric Association and many other professional and lay organizations gave testimony in the hearings that he held to gather information (N. Stotland, February 1988, unpublished testimony). After hearing all of the testimony, Koop declined to produce the requested formal report, concluding instead that there was insufficient evidence to conclude that abortion has negative effects and that a comprehensive, broad-based, longitudinal research project on the reproductive lives of women is indicated. There is much we do not know about the biological, social, and psychological forces that shape women's reproductive lives and experiences.

We also do not know what lies ahead. It is likely that access to abortion will be decided legislatively, state by state and district by district. Restrictions may be enacted under the guise of mandates that have an emotional appeal to some people—for example, as requirements to inform or obtain consent from a woman's husband or an adolescent's parents. A spousal notification law was passed by the legislature and signed into law by the governor of Pennsylvania in the fall of 1989 (Pennsylvania Senate Bill 369). Such restrictions pose specific problems for the psychiatrist involved in a pregnant woman's care. They short-circuit the therapeutic evolution of a patient's decision to inform her spouse or parents, overlook the fact that some spouses and parents do not have benevolent relationships with pregnant patients, and deprive patients of autonomy in decisions that will be played out in their own bodies.

A generation of citizens has grown up and a generation of psychiatrists and other physicians has been trained in the decade and a half since *Roe v. Wade*. Most of them regard abortion as a fact of life—a legitimate, though painful, option in a crisis. They have not experienced medical or psychiatric practice without that option. Most have been trained with the belief that the responsibility and privilege for medical decision making lies primarily with the patient. The doctor is seen as a source of information and insight, a performer of technical procedures, and a provider of emotional support. A changed governmental stance and agenda will force physicians to reexamine the relationship among reproductive psychology and choice, abortion, and psychiatry. Abortion is no longer a taboo subject, but it may well become a limited reality.

Since the *Roe v. Wade* decision, most laypersons have not had to give much thought to reproductive choice. State laws restricting abortion were regularly passed by legislators going through the motions to satisfy antichoice components of their constituencies, knowing that these statutes would be overturned at the state or national Supreme Court level. The U.S. Congress did outlaw federal funding of abortions (Annas 1989). Now, the necessity for advocates of choice—noninterference by government—with regard to abortion to declare themselves and join the legislative process if access is to be maintained may result in new alignments and other unimagined consequences. Varying state regulations, facilities, and prices may engender geographic abortion traffic. Women may resort to illegal procedures, as they did (by the millions) in the past. It is important to remember that there is no developed culture described now or in history in which the practice of abortion was successfully eliminated. Abortion could only have been proscribed in the Hippocratic oath if people knew about and performed it. Obviously, women all over the world throughout history have felt sufficiently desperate to terminate pregnancies that they risked their lives to do so (Cook and Dickens 1978). It is reasonable to assume that in North America in the future, as in the past, the affluent, knowledgeable, and sophisticated will manage to obtain the medically adequate services that they desire while the poor, weak, and uneducated will go without (Berger 1978; Tietze 1984).

Fundamental Realities

The American Public Health Association estimated that, before the legalization of abortion in the United States, at least one million women per year had illegal abortions. In 1965, before abortion was decriminalized, 235

(20%) of all deaths related to pregnancy and childbirth were also related to abortion. Many other women suffered severe medical complications, surgery, and sterility. The number decreased by approximately 90% after legalization. The following statistics have been reported by the U.S. Centers for Disease Control and the National Center for Health Statistics (1989). There are .5 deaths per 100,000 abortions. The risk of dying from medical abortion is one-twenty-fifth or less of that of carrying a pregnancy to term, which is a pregnant woman's only alternative, and one-one-hundredth the risk of major surgery. The mortality rate from tonsillectomy is twice as high. The risk of serious complications of first-trimester abortion is less than one-half of 1%. Rape and incest are frequently discussed in connection with unwanted pregnancy and abortion. It has been calculated that one woman in three will be raped or sexually abused in her lifetime and that 5% of rapes result in pregnancy. One in 10 U.S. women becomes pregnant during her high school years. Teenage women abort 42% of their pregnancies; of these women, 96% are unmarried. Seventy percent of women obtaining abortions are white, 57% are nulliparous, 90% are in their first trimester of pregnancy (half in the first 8 weeks), and 61% are having their first abortion. Less than 1% of abortions are performed after 20 weeks. Ninety percent of abortions are performed by cervical dilatation and suction curettage, requiring a little more than 10 minutes, under local anesthesia.

Most abortions take place outside general hospitals. There is no evidence that early abortions performed in hospitals are safer than those in outpatient clinics or doctors' offices. The latter cost about $213, about one-third the price of a hospital abortion; however, these facilities and hospitals willing to perform significant numbers of (or even any) abortions are few and unevenly distributed. Thirty percent of women live in counties without any abortion provider; this includes 82% of all U.S. counties. These women undergo far fewer abortions.

Psychiatric Questions and Misconceptions

The issue of access to abortion has been framed in affectively loaded and factually inaccurate language. Much of this language has become part of the popular parlance; however, psychiatrists are aware that language carries emotional and connotational baggage with it even when such meanings are not part of the conscious intention of those who use the terms. For example, opponents of access to abortion call themselves "pro-life," linguistically preempting humanistic values and intentions for their point of view and restricting the focus on human life to the embryo. One of the core issues articulated in the U.S. Supreme Court *Webster v. Reproductive Health Services* (1989) decision is the question of fetal "personhood" (Annas 1989). Although the federal government has yielded to and acted on this limited view, funds for research and services in the areas of contraception, prenatal care, and maternal and child health have been slashed rather than increased. Similarly, groups opposed to abortion have characterized their opponents as "pro-abortion." But abortion is a procedure. There is no question of promoting this procedure per se, and no one does. The issues are privacy, autonomy, choice, emancipation for reproductively driven strictures, gender equity, and personal and family well-being. The designations *anti-choice* and *pro-choice* are the only ones that convey the viewpoints accurately.

Even in the absence of governmental restrictions, abortion raises fundamental issues in psychiatric research and clinical practice. Why do men and women conceive pregnancies that one or both then decide are untenable? Do contraceptives fail? Are people dissuaded from using them by adverse scientific findings and sensationalized court cases concerning gruesome complications? Does contraceptive use conflict with powerful psychosocial forces, such as the need to prove gender adequacy by conception or gender domination by exposing a partner to pregnancy or the aversion to the conscious admission of sexual intentions by making contraceptive preparations (Tietze 1975)? We understand very little about the psychodynamics and psychobiology of the wish to conceive, bear, and care for children.

This brings us to a fundamental reality of abortion. Abortion is often discussed as though it were an isolated decision and procedure. But abortion only becomes an issue when pregnancy has been conceived and experienced as unmanageable by a concerned party. This is a major psychosocial crisis. A decision about abortion is always made in the context of that existing crisis (Shusterman 1976). The sequelae of legal abortion must always be compared with the sequelae of the only other options available— illegal abortion and childbearing. Unplanned or unwanted conception constitutes a biopsychosocial failure and deciding what to do about it is an emotionally wrenching process. Abortion is one possible outcome of that decision, and it can never be understood out of that context.

Under what conditions did the conception occur? Were the man and woman ignorant of the biology of conception? Why? Why does the sexual passion of the moment overwhelm the judgment of some people at some times and not those of others at other times? Were they overwhelmed by social circumstances—such as poverty, abuse, and discrimination—that diminished their real and perceived capacity to make or implement reproductive decisions? Were they unable to discuss or manage the allotment of responsibility for the outcome of intercourse between them? Paradoxically, a woman overwhelmed by the care of children already born may be less able to obtain contraceptive care and insist on conditions for sexual contact with men than a woman less familiar with the realities of procreation and parenthood.

Another misconception is that the availability of abortion, by itself, confers reproductive freedom on women. As the questions just posed indicate,

reproductive behavior is interwoven into a dense fabric of cultural traditions, social circumstances, family expectations, and individual medical
and psychological needs. Reproduction is fraught with tremendous psychological meaning for members of both sexes. It is one of life's organizing
goals and one of life's most awesome and consuming responsibilities. Even
where contraception and abortion are widely available, most people choose
to have and care for children. What does the term *freedom* mean in this
context? It is a much richer and more complicated freedom than the right
to choose a college major or cosmetic surgery, although even those choices
are not completely free. For one woman, it means the freedom to end a
pregnancy that she finds inconvenient or impossible; for another, it means
the freedom to bear and care for as many children as she can conceive or
simply to continue one current, highly desired pregnancy. Freedom can
be constrained as a result of pressure on a woman either to continue a
gestation she does not want or to end one that is inconvenient for someone
else. The other person may be her male partner, her parent, her employer,
or anyone else whose feelings, opinions, and power are significant in her
life. Successful reproduction, which may be the outcome a woman desires,
requires substantial environmental support. The absence of any or all components of that support constrains a woman's reproductive freedom.

Many clinical situations, particularly those in which psychiatrists may become involved, are even more complicated. The following is a clinical example.

> Psychiatric consultation was sought by the gynecology service for a 23-year-old
> woman pregnant for the third time. She had children 1 and 2 years of age and
> was at 8 weeks' gestation. The patient was mentally retarded, with a mental age
> of 3 years. She and her children lived under the care of her mother, who was
> barely able to cope and who felt that another pregnancy and delivery and the
> birth of a third child would be injurious to herself, her daughter (the patient),
> and her daughter's existing children. She could not control the patient's behavior
> and movements; the patient was impregnated by unknown men in the neigh-
> borhood. She was able to feed and toilet herself, but her hygiene was poor. At
> the time of her second delivery, she panicked; unable to cooperate with the
> obstetrician, she sustained a fourth-degree perineal laceration that became in-
> fected because of her inability to keep the area clean. She required readmission
> to the hospital for a major revision of the wound under general anesthesia. At
> the time of psychiatric consultation, she was unable to remember and repeat the
> names of her children, her address, or the date. Although her level of compre-
> hension was limited, she indicated that she did not want to have an abortion.
> What action would express this woman's freedom?

Values: Understanding the Realities of Reproductive Responsibility and Women's Lives

In our society, the overwhelming responsibility for and performance of
child care resides with mothers. Women also assume the majority of care

of ill and disabled adults in their families. Although environmental supports are vital, no social agency or cultural tradition has significantly modified that predominant role. The majority of active fathers rear children in households where a woman assumes the managerial, long-range planning, emotional, and hands-on aspects of care. Most single parents are mothers who receive no financial support from the fathers of their children. So, too, to a woman who has conceived falls the responsibility to decide about her capacity to gestate, bear, and care for a child. If she has a child or children, she bears the responsibility for their ongoing care before and after the birth of another child. No one else has a greater knowledge of or stake in her children's needs and well-being and the probable effects of an additional pregnancy and family member on family function. The gestation and birth of a child can take place only as an integral function of a woman's body. Here, too, no single option or behavior constitutes freedom. A woman may feel that an abortion is a terrifying and repugnant intrusion on her body and her nascent relationship with the fetus but that she has a moral responsibility to undergo the procedure in the interests of others to whom she has a superseding responsibility that no one else will assume.

Perspectives: Scientific, Religious, Legal, Anthropological, Social, Racial, Gender

Various perspectives can be brought to bear on the specific clinical problems and populations psychiatrists face when induced abortion is an issue. What are the data? And what are the difficulties in gathering and interpreting them? Susan Blumenthal reviews the literature in Chapter 2. As mentioned before, some authors before the 1970s studied adverse sequelae after abortion. Some women felt guilty; a small percentage suffered major psychiatric illness. There has been no way to make the studies double-blind or meaningfully control them. The values and expectations of the investigators also color the methods and conclusions. Patients cannot be randomly assigned either to become pregnant or to undergo abortion or delivery. It is reasonable to assume that the factors that make unintended or undesired pregnancy more likely also increase the risk of psychological symptoms after it occurs. Studies performed after abortion became legal demonstrated fewer or no adverse sequelae.

The sociolegal climate in which abortion occurs can only be controlled in historical or cross-cultural studies. These studies can also highlight culturally linked assumptions about psychiatric concomitants of abortion. We have been unable to locate any studies from countries where abortion is widely performed indicating significant adverse outcomes compared with other alternatives. Studies from two European countries indicate that children born after their mothers were refused abortion did not fare as well in society as case-matched control subjects (Forssman and Thuwe 1981; Matejcek et al. 1978). In the United States, longitudinal follow-up of any group of patients after a medical procedure is uncommon and difficult because of the lack of centralized medical record keeping. Research and treatment are also hampered by the fact that the reproductive status of women seen in psychiatric outpatient and inpatient settings is often over-looked or not reported. Recent abortion or delivery may be buried in a woman's history rather than highlighted as a possible factor in her illness and decision to seek psychiatric care. Psychiatric and gynecologic specialists tend to function within circumscribed areas of concern and intervention.

Despite these difficulties, there is a useful literature on psychiatric out-come of induced abortion. Compared with parturition, abortion is asso-ciated with a lower incidence of psychiatric illness and hospitalization (Brewer 1977). Risk factors for psychiatric sequelae include prior psychiatric illness, psychosocial stress, and an abortion decision brought about by external pressure (Moseley et al. 1981). The impact of values and expectations on the scientific work is evident because only some of the newer studies included attempts to reveal positive sequelae. Many women reported that the process of thinking through and following through the abortion de-cision was positive. In addition to the relief they experienced after the problem pregnancy had ended, they felt that they had learned another level of responsibility for and control of their lives. Observations from other cultures indicate that the same conflicts and ambivalence are present. For example, in Japan one goddess is believed to take an interest in small children. At shrines dedicated to her, infant bibs and toys donated by bereaved parents are hung. Among those making the donations are women who have undergone abortions. Abortions are commonly used in Japan to limit family size. The donation to the shrine does not necessarily imply regret, but it does suggest a wish to set the soul of the abortus at rest so that it will not make trouble for the woman.

Law is humanity's way of codifying morality and regulating society. Many people believe that abortion was illegal everywhere and in every historical era until the *Roe v. Wade* decision. It is also common to believe that most organized religions have been and continue to be opposed to abortion. The history of abortion law reveals, however, that the outlawing of abortion is a relatively new phenomenon. For most of the history of the Roman Catholic Church, Catholic law held that a fetus did not have a soul until some weeks into gestation. Quickening, the perception of fetal move-ments by a pregnant woman, was used as a limit for centuries. Most major religious groups other than the Roman Catholic Church have adopted an active stance in favor of reproductive choice, including abortion as an option. The outlawing of abortion in the United States was part of the medicalization of obstetric and gynecologic care in the late nineteenth and early twentieth centuries. There was a concerted attempt to portray lay midwifery as dangerous, and abortion was one of the services midwives performed.

Particular Populations

Psychiatrists in practice must be aware of the implications of abortion in various situations and populations. During discussion of a patient's sexual practices, a psychiatrist may become aware that the issue of possible or probable conception is not being dealt with. What leads the patient to choose a particular contraceptive method or none? Does the patient have a conscious or unconscious reason for wanting to conceive a pregnancy that, if it occurs, will cause unmanageable problems in her life? Or are there other problems with contraception that overshadow the patient's concern about pregnancy? She may have a partner who insists on proving his virility by impregnation. Many men, especially in the era of oral contraceptives, have come to regard contraception as a woman's responsibility. They refuse to use condoms, making a woman choose among the relationship, the risks of other methods, and an unwanted pregnancy. Women in conflict about the morality of sexual intercourse sometimes believe that contraceptive preparations underscore their intent to engage in this forbidden activity. It is more psychologically acceptable to be "swept off one's feet." This is particularly true of adolescents.

Adolescents share several other attributes relevant to abortion contexts and decisions. Their impulsivity and difficulty conceptualizing the long-term effects of current behavior impair their ability to control sexual impulses and use contraception effectively. Young adolescents do not have a realistic understanding of parenthood. They may become pregnant in competition with their mothers, or conceive in hope of having a baby who will love them. Adolescents from troubled families have an increased risk of unplanned pregnancy, poor pregnancy outcome, and difficulties with parenting. The same immaturity and psychological conflicts affect the adolescent as she makes decisions about a pregnancy. She may suppress her awareness of the delivery that is inevitable in several months and focus instead on her fear of an abortion procedure in the immediate future. She may also be so panicked at the thought of labor or motherhood that she cannot draw on available resources to plan to maintain a pregnancy that she wants. Her male partner is likely to be young and overwhelmed as well.

The involvement of parents is complicated. The parents of adolescent mothers may be called on to play a role in the care of both mother and child. They know their daughter and the family values and religion. They can also exert tremendous pressure on a young woman. They have their own preferences and agendas. In the last analysis and according to the available data, the adolescent who becomes a mother usually becomes the primary and permanent caretaker for her child. Her education and employment opportunities are severely and usually permanently curtailed, and her child is at risk for prematurity and other perinatal complications, neglect, poor school performance, and many other negative outcomes. Relatively few adolescent mothers relinquish children for adoption.

An adolescent's ignorance, denial, and dread of confronting her parents with the revelation of her pregnancy may delay a decision about abortion to the middle trimester. Later abortions are more complex surgical procedures and are associated with a higher risk of adverse psychiatric sequelae. This association may be secondary to the fact that women with psychiatric and psychosocial problems delay the acknowledgment and diagnosis of pregnancy and the decision to abort. Additional complicating factors are the fact that the pregnancy has become public knowledge and that the abortion may be difficult to obtain.

Second-trimester abortions can also be stressful to gynecologic or abortion clinic staff members. Psychiatrists may be called on to consult with staffs or individual care providers. Dealing on a daily basis with patients who have decided to terminate pregnancies is a challenge. Some patients appreciate a great deal of hands-on support, whereas others cope by suppressing their feelings until the procedure has been completed and they have returned home. Medical staff members must try to determine and respond to the needs of each individual. Although they obtain gratification from helping women to resolve the crisis of problematic pregnancies and they focus on providing that care, terminating pregnancies was not the goal for which most health care providers aimed when they began their training. It is, at best, a sad solution to a failure of some kind. Later abortions may entail a labor process, causing more pain to the patient. A second-trimester or late first-trimester abortion, depending on the procedure employed, confronts staff members with the sight of recognizable fetal parts or whole embryos. This is a stressful experience. Staff discussions, the recognition of the relief of suffering for the patients involved, and consultation with a mental health professional help staff members to cope.

There are particular issues concerning black women and abortion. Black women are more likely to be poor and, therefore, to have less access to contraceptive, antenatal, and abortion services than white women. Restrictive laws often specifically target facilities and services funded by public moneys. Some black community leaders have indicated that they believe that access to abortion for black women is provided by the white establishment in an attempt to minimize the increase in the black population; the term *genocide* has been used. Women who are educationally disadvantaged may invest more of their identity in motherhood, because employment opportunities are few. In some black subpopulations, adolescent pregnancy and parenting are modal. There may be more social and religious sentiment against abortion than against unwed motherhood. The number of adoptive homes for black children is insufficient to meet the need. A movement in a past decade to foster cross-racial adoption has fallen into disfavor. Lately, some social agencies have reexamined the requirements for foster and adoptive families to determine whether they conflicted needlessly with black subcommunity norms.

Another group with an important perspective on abortion is men. In one sense, men are irrelevant to the abortion decision and procedure that intrinsically concern a woman's body and future. But men are also progenitors of the problem pregnancy. Sometimes a man is construed as the villain who impregnated a woman against her will, before the age of majority, or without concern for outcome, leaving the woman to make the decision and bear and care for the child or undergo an abortion. Some men pressure or expect their partners to have abortions because they do not wish to enter a committed relationship or assume responsibility for a child. But many men have profound feelings about pregnancy, abortion, and their own responsibility and exclusion. In the decision-making process or their own psychotherapy, they may display guilt, rage, and feelings of helplessness and loss, or they may experience the abortion decision and process as a maturational step, a commitment to limit or delay reproduction until maturation and circumstances allow for a more gratifying and responsible fatherhood. A woman's current pregnancy may be her partner's only or long-awaited opportunity to become a father. Her abortion may represent an act of rage and destruction against him. The role and rights of the potential father are an issue in the legislative and judicial process. Male partners have sought injunctions to prevent women from obtaining desired abortions.

Another group whose interest in abortion has been highlighted by laws proposed in several states is the parents of young women who are pregnant. Antiabortion advocates have introduced and enacted legislation requiring parental notification or consent for abortions performed on women younger then the age of majority. The idea of spousal and parental participation in decisions about pregnancy has a certain commonsense appeal. A pregnant woman's partner and the parents of a pregnant minor girl have a biological relationship to the embryo and a close emotional relationship to the pregnant woman. Under optimal and even average circumstances, the husband or parents are the woman's confidants, psychosocial supports, and advisers. Why should notification and consent require legal intervention? The issue only arises when the normative or ideal relationships do not exist. Then, the pregnant woman does not perceive her husband or parents as potentially helpful as she makes her decision. They may be psychologically or geographically removed, doctrinaire, self-centered, hostile, or even physically threatening. The adolescent who does not wish to tell her parents that she is pregnant and plans to have an abortion typically fears exile from the family home. Such situations can sometimes be resolved by family intervention, but the contested laws do not mandate family financial support or fund individual or family counseling, as they might if they were truly intended to facilitate supported choice. The legislation formalizes the ultimate control of the husband, family, and state of a woman's decision about her pregnancy and interpolates bureaucratic procedures to complicate and deter access to abortion.

Psychiatric Implications of Recent Changes in Abortion Law

Recent changes in the response of the U.S. Supreme Court to state abortion legislation are likely to have direct and indirect effects on psychiatric practice. Women experiencing pregnancies they find untenable and lacking access to legal and safe abortion will be under tremendous stress. The fact that a once-legal procedure has been denied to them may result in significant disaffection and bitterness. Those injured by traumatic and unsafe abortions performed by themselves or other unqualified persons will be at risk for posttraumatic stress disorders and other psychiatric illness. Women may be constrained to remain in physically or psychologically abusive relationships that have resulted in undesired pregnancy.

Psychiatry and the subject of abortion will interface directly in several clinical situations. Preexisting major psychiatric illness is one. Psychiatrists are confronted with patients who have suffered major postpartum psychiatric decompensations after previous deliveries and who, at serious risk of recurrence, consult them for advice. Other patients suffer from chronic psychiatric diseases that make them unable to care for children. In some cases, the tenuous ability to care for one or more existing children would be severely threatened by the birth of another baby. In others, the mother has lost custody of several children, who usually remain in state guardianship and without permanent parental arrangements. The loss of custody is also extremely painful and disabling for the patient. Lack of access to abortion consigns such a patient to the continuation of another pregnancy, a delivery, and another loss, with deleterious effects on both mother and child.

The administration of psychotropic medication is another complicating clinical issue. Psychiatrists may, in emergency situations, prescribe agents with unknown or adverse effects on embryonic development before a patient's pregnancy can be diagnosed. The Missouri law upheld by the Supreme Court in the *Webster* case severely restricts or prevents the expenditure of public funds to counsel or encourage a woman to have an abortion unless it is necessary to save her life. This could mean that a psychiatrist in a hospital receiving any public funding would be forbidden to discuss abortion as an option with such a patient. Investigators from the government or from antiabortion groups might appear in clinical settings to determine whether the law was being obeyed.

Before the *Roe v. Wade* decision, and under the new Missouri (*Webster*) law upheld by the Supreme Court, a threat to a woman's life was often the only accepted criterion for abortion. Psychiatrists were frequently called on to evaluate suicidality in pregnant women seeking the termination of pregnancy. As mentioned before, such assessments are inherently complicated by the constrained circumstances under which they occur. In addition, they raise problems that have become more focused by changes in the legal and social climate since *Roe v. Wade*. In this litigious era, will psychiatrists be willing to draw and document diagnostic conclusions on the basis of insufficient evidence? Criteria for suicidality for pregnant women may be compared with those for involuntary commitment for suicide risk. Will we implicitly or explicitly instruct patients to tell us that they have made previous attempts, have the means at hand, have family histories of suicide, or have major disturbances of impulse control or mood? Will we be willing to defend our opinions and recommendations in the context of peer review, professional regulation bodies, and courts of law?

What will be the implications for a woman who obtains an abortion on grounds of suicidality? Many more women are active in public and corporate life than in the past. Since social support for the combination of maternal and career responsibilities has not increased, women with major educational and career aspirations will be among those who seek to terminate pregnancies that threaten to undermine important plans and who are sophisticated enough to obtain psychiatric consultation for the purpose. Psychiatric and medical confidentiality are frequently abrogated in such contexts as political campaigns, and psychiatric contact and illness still, unfortunately, carry significant stigma. How will an assessment of suicidality, made by a psychiatrist trying to help a patient, affect the patient's future ability to realize her goals and capacities and to make a contribution to society?

Another important clinical implication of the new rulings is the assertion of the state's vested interest in the life of the fetus. This policy logically leads to government-ordered forced obstetrical interventions in situations in which some party alleges that a procedure the mother has refused would be in the interests of the fetus. There are clinical situations in which physicians' investments in good obstetrical outcome are severely tried by a pregnant woman's noncompliance with medically advised behavior. It is extremely painful to care for a neonate suffering drug withdrawal or to watch a pregnant woman chain-smoke. But forcing interventions on a woman in the interest of her unborn child leads to unacceptable and socially ineffective outcomes. For example, women have been convicted of child abuse for substance use during pregnancy. Is there clinical evidence that such a policy is an effective deterrent or treatment for substance abuse? Will a child fare better because its mother has been incarcerated? In clinical practice, a state may intervene in psychiatrists' and patients' decisions to use psychotropic medication during pregnancy or force psychiatrists to involuntarily hospitalize women whose antepartum behavior is not in compliance with state or obstetrical guidelines. Paradoxically, breaching the boundary of a woman's decision-making power over her body opens the door to state-mandated abortions as well.

Conclusion

Abortion and the recent added constraints on choice have profound implications for psychiatrists. Psychiatrists and their organizations are sources for scientific and clinical information about psychiatric issues in abortion— for governmental bodies, medical and mental health colleagues, and the press. Unwanted pregnancy may result from psychosocial conflict or frank psychiatric illness. A woman in conflict about a pregnancy, her male partner, and her family may benefit from psychiatric intervention in the decision-making process and as they cope with whatever decision they make. Issues involving abortion are factors in psychotherapy with men and women. Psychiatric illness and treatment often complicate decision making about pregnancy, and pregnancy complicates decision making about psychiatric treatment. Specific populations—such as minority men and women, women undergoing second-trimester abortion, and adolescents—have characteristic issues about which psychiatrists need to be knowledgeable. Psychiatrists must examine and manage the values, beliefs, and feelings about abortion that they bring to the public and clinical setting.

Changes in laws governing abortion have far-reaching implications for psychiatrists and their patients. In the words of George Annas (1989):

> A majority of the Supreme Court, for the first time in two decades, is willing to discuss abortion rights without reference to the rights of individual women or the rights of their physicians. This could have implications for birth-control measures other than abortion that act after fertilization, as well as for other areas of medical practice, such as the patient's right to refuse treatment. . . . Thus, the abortion debate has returned to the political arena, where it has been consistently impossible to resolve. In states that decide to add restrictions on abortion, physicians and their pregnant patients may find their medical and moral options sharply limited. (p. 1202)

References

Annas GJ: The Supreme Court, privacy, and abortion. N Engl J Med 321:1200–1203,1989

Ashton JR: The psychosocial outcome of induced abortion. Br J Ob Gyn 87:1115–1122, 1980

Berger LR: Abortions in America: the effects of restrictive funding. N Engl J Med 298:1474–1477, 1978

Bolter S: The psychiatrist's role in therapeutic abortion: the unwitting accomplice. Am J Psychiatry 119:312–316, 1962

Brewer C: Incidence of post-abortion psychosis: a prospective study. Br Med J 1:476–477, 1977

Cook RJ, Dickens BM: A decade of international change in abortion law: 1967–1977. Am J Public Health 68:637–644, 1978

David HP, Rasmussen NK, Holst E: Postpartum and postabortion psychotic reactions. Fam Plann Perspect 13:88–92, 1981

Ewing JA, Rouse BA: Therapeutic abortion and a prior psychiatric history. Am J Psychiatry 130:37–40, 1973

Ford C, Atkinson R, Bugonier J: Therapeutic abortion: who needs a psychiatrist? Obstet Gynecol 38:206–213, 1971a

Ford C, Castelnuova-Tedesca P, Long I: Is abortion a therapeutic procedure in psychiatry? JAMA 218:1173–1178, 1971b

Forssman H, Thuwe I: Continued follow-up study of 120 persons born after refusal of application for therapeutic abortion. Acta Psychiatr Scand 64:142–149, 1981

Friedman CM, Greenspan R, Mittleman F: The decision-making process and the outcome of therapeutic abortion. Am J Psychiatry 131:1332–1337, 1974

Matejcek A, Dytrych Z, Schuller V: Children from unwanted pregnancies. Acta Psychiatr Scand 57:67–90, 1978

Moseley DT, Follingstad DR, Harley H: Psychological factors that predict reaction to abortion. J Clin Psychol 37:276–279, 1981

Pasnau RO: Psychiatric complications of therapeutic abortion. Obstet Gynecol 40:252–256, 1972

Roe v. Wade, 410 U.S. 113 (1973)

Senay E: Therapeutic abortion. Arch Gen Psychiatry 23:408–415, 1970

Shusterman LR: The psychosocial factors of the abortion experience: a critical review. Psychology of Women Quarterly 1:79–102, 1976

Tietze C: Contraceptive practice in the context of a non-restrictive abortion law. Fam Plann Perspect 7:197–202, 1975

Tietze C: The public health effects of legal abortion in the United States. Fam Plann Perspect 16:26–28, 1984

U.S. Centers for Disease Control, National Center for Health Statistics, as quoted in Public Health Policy Implications of Abortion. Washington, DC, The American College of Obstetricians and Gynecologists, 1990

Webster v. Reproductive Health Services, 109 S Ct 3040 (1989)

Chapter 2

Psychiatric Consequences of Abortion: Overview of Research Findings

Susan J. Blumenthal, M.D., M.P.A.

In recent years, increasing controversy has surrounded the issue of abortion. In particular, the U.S. Supreme Court *Webster v. Reproductive Health Services* (1989) decision and the unpublished 1989 report of U.S. Surgeon General C. Everett Koop on the public health effects of abortion have prompted a reexamination of the medical and psychiatric impact of this procedure. The nation's attention has been turned once again to this emotionally charged issue that has been argued anew by each generation throughout history (Surgeon General's Report 1989). The debate centers on the fundamental choice between competing rights: the government's right to protect human life and a woman's right to make one of the most important decisions in her life—whether and when to have a child. It was just 16 years before that the Supreme Court (*Doe v. Bolton* 1973; *Roe v. Wade* 1973) decided that a woman's rights under the U.S. Constitution included the right to have an abortion. This determination was based on the court's interpretation of the Fourteenth Amendment to the Constitution, which held that a fetus is not a person and, therefore, is not guaranteed the same rights as women.

Before the liberalization of the abortion laws in 1973, abortions were illegal in all states except to preserve the life of the mother. Therefore, abortions were performed for "therapeutic" reasons, including medical or psychiatric indications. Medical reasons for pregnancy termination included illnesses such as heart disease, kidney failure, malignancy, and abdominal emergencies (Shusterman 1976). As physicians' abilities to prevent many health risks associated with pregnancy increased, psychiatric problems became the primary indication for abortion. This indication was broadly interpreted, with the criteria varying from hospital to hospital (Nadelson 1972). This standard persisted until 1973 when the need for a therapeutic reason was dropped with the legalization of abortion.

Numerous explanations have been cited in the literature as reasons for unwanted pregnancies, including rape, incest, denial of or refusal to recognize the possibility of getting pregnant, contraceptive failure, unconscious motivations, and role redefinition. In addition, adolescent pregnancy has become an increasing problem in the United States. Young women may become pregnant without being in a stable relationship and often are not emotionally or financially prepared to care for a child adequately. Other women who unintentionally become pregnant may wish to fulfill education or career plans. Older married women may seek abortions to prevent the expansion of their family. In most cases, the motivations for seeking an abortion are strongly felt and, in part, these reasons may protect against what might otherwise be an experience of loss or regret (Surgeon General's Report 1989).

Legalized abortion has permitted a woman to decide whether and when she will have a child and to make that decision with societal sanction (Friedman et al. 1974). Furthermore, the legalization of the procedure and technical advances improving the safety of medical technology have resulted in a reduction in mortality rates from the procedure; childbirth now carries a greater risk of morbidity and mortality than does a therapeutic abortion (Henshaw 1986; Nadelson and Notman 1984). As a result, abortion has become a safe and effective method for a woman with an unwanted pregnancy to resolve an overwhelming personal crisis.

The recent resurgence of controversy surrounding abortion has again raised questions about the safety of abortion and its long-term effects on women's physical health and mental health. In this chapter, I review the research literature on the psychiatric sequelae of abortion and discuss the methodological problems that complicate interpretation of findings from these studies. I also review predictors of difficulty after abortion and the relationship of having an abortion to the development of subsequent psychiatric illness. Additionally, I compare the consequences of having an abortion with those of carrying through an unwanted pregnancy. I conclude the chapter by presenting some implications of the literature for clinical practice and recommendations for future studies in this area.

Methodological Issues

Although the research literature on abortion includes observations on several hundred thousand patients for many years, the interpretation of this body of evidence is difficult. In part, this is because articles on abortion have taken many forms, including clinical case reports, personal opinions, reviews, commentaries, surveys, and systematic research studies. Only a few of these reports, however, can withstand rigorous scrutiny of their research design. In her excellent and comprehensive review of the literature, Shusterman (1976) detailed many of the methodological problems that have complicated research on abortion. For example, in experimental studies, the outcome of the effects of the procedure are often measured by comparing groups that differ either in certain initial characteristics or in the procedure to which they are subjected. Unfortunately, less than 10% of studies of the psychiatric effects of abortion reported in the literature make use of a control or comparison group. Several of the studies suffer because they have small or poorly defined samples, lacking information on subjects who chose not to participate in the study. Others are flawed because the length of time between the abortion and the assessment of outcome was too variable.

Research on abortion conducted from the 1940s through the 1960s generally was poorly designed, had severe methodological problems, and appeared to be influenced by investigator bias, whereas later studies that addressed some of these design concerns produced more reliable data. Particular problems in the early research were a lack of specification of the type, severity, or frequency of the psychological complication studied. In addition, investigators often did not use any standardized method to evaluate psychiatric symptoms.

Various methods have been used in these studies to assess the psychological status of patients before and after therapeutic abortion. Interviews and questions are most common. In many of the studies, however, the methods are not well described and demographic variables may not be considered. In retrospective studies, some patients were interviewed soon after their abortions; others were interviewed much later either by telephone or directly (Shusterman 1976). There is a lack of consensus on symptoms, severity, and duration of mental disorder as well as an absence of careful screening for psychiatric history. Furthermore, most interviews in these studies were conducted by males, with no consideration given to the effects of the interviewer's sex on the response of the woman being interviewed. According to Kummer (1963), data collected on a topic as sensitive as abortion may differ in type and interpretation when collected by male and female researchers. In addition, attempts at objective behavioral assessments are rare in these studies. When these assessments are attempted, the methods used are often of unknown reliability or validity. An additional limitation of many of the investigations has been the self-selection of the sample. Women whose abortions are performed by private physicians are not represented and are estimated to compose about 4% of cases.

Some of the reports do not differentiate among results from therapeutic, illegal, and requested abortions, where the emotional context and indications may be quite variable. Studies performed in other countries that have different cultural mores may yield outcomes different from those in studies undertaken in the United States, making cross-cultural comparisons difficult. Furthermore, the high cost and logistical problems associated with longitudinal research make longer-term prospective studies difficult to undertake.

Despite the relative methodological ease of clearly defining onset of psychiatric symptoms after the termination of a pregnancy, few epidemiological studies of postabortion psychiatric sequelae have been conducted. There has been general resistance in the field to viewing postpartum or postabortion psychiatric disorders as distinct clinical conditions with symptoms, psychopathology, and a prognosis that differ from the well-described mental illnesses (David et al. 1981). In this regard, the DSM-III-R of the American Psychiatric Association (1987) does not have a separate category for postpartum mental disorders.

As a result of many of the methodological problems just described, the literature on the psychological impact of induced abortion is often contradictory. Most of the papers on this subject were written between 1945 and 1980. Few recent reports on this issue exist. Nevertheless, a critical review of the systematic research studies conducted to date yields the conclusion that there are few psychiatric sequelae from the procedure. It is rare for a study to conclude that there are severe psychological consequences. Several of the studies find that the consequences vary with other factors. Some investigators suggest that because of divergent results found in the literature, the psychological effects of abortion are unknown (Shusterman 1976). In this chapter, I highlight some of the pertinent studies on abortion. Readers are encouraged to consult other excellent reviews of this subject for more in-depth coverage (Doane and Quigley 1981; Gould 1980; Handy 1982; Nadelson 1972; Osofsky and Osofsky 1972; Pasnau 1972; Schusterman 1976; Walter 1970; Whittington 1970). Unfortunately, few recent studies or reviews have been conducted on this subject (Adler et al. 1990).

Psychiatric Consequences of Abortion

As mentioned before, the findings on the psychiatric impact of abortion are contradictory, in part because of the methodological flaws in the research. Moreover, findings from the literature on illegal, therapeutic, and legal abortion must be examined separately, because the emotional and social contexts of abortions vary greatly depending on the way in which the procedures and the women requesting them are viewed by society (Shusterman 1976). Psychological responses after an abortion reflect the scope of emotions that accompany experiencing and resolving an unwanted pregnancy (Adler et al. 1990). Although studies reveal feelings of regret, sadness, or guilt, the bulk of scientific literature indicates that legal abortion of an unwanted pregnancy in the first trimester does not pose psychological complications for most women (Adler et al. 1990).

1940–1960: Early Studies of Abortion

One of the earliest reviews of the effects of therapeutic abortion was a study conducted by Hesseltine et al. (1940). These investigators reviewed the psychiatric records of 82 women for 1–8 years after the women had therapeutic abortions and found satisfactory or improved outcomes in 21 subjects, unchanged outcomes in 22, unsatisfactory outcomes in 3, and undertermined outcomes in 35. Despite their findings of generally satisfactory outcomes, the authors concluded that abortions were rarely necessary. This perplexing conclusion and the methodological problems in the study (such as the manner by which psychiatric examinations were performed, the reasons for the many undetermined outcomes, and the elapsed time from procedure to assessment) make the study of little value to our understanding of the psychiatric impact of the procedure (Shusterman 1976).

Hamilton (1940) evaluated the period of time between therapeutic, illegal, and spontaneous abortion and its emotional impact. In this study, only 30 of the 537 women interviewed had obtained therapeutic abortions, whereas the remainder of the sample had spontaneous or illegal abortions. Forty-six percent of the women in the sample experienced regret, 39% felt relief, and 15% were indifferent after the procedure. The women who obtained an illegal or therapeutic abortion experienced the least regret. The author concluded that the emotional impact of abortion was minimal. Hamilton (1941) reinterviewed 100 women from the 1940 study and concluded that with time, regretful feelings were replaced with feelings of relief and satisfaction. Since distinctions were not made between the types of abortions in the study or between the methods of psychiatric evaluation, the results of this investigation are difficult to interpret.

Ebaugh and Hesuer (1947) evaluated 47 women after abortions and found that feelings of guilt, self-deprecation, and hostility toward their male partners developed after the procedure. Methodological flaws make it difficult to interpret the conclusions of this study.

Wilson and Caine (1951) investigated the psychiatric sequelae after an abortion in women who had received the procedure in a particular facility between 1930 and 1949. Despite interviewing only nine women who reported minor difficulties, such as some feelings of guilt, the authors concluded that abortion had deep and lasting emotional effects. In a subsequent study of 25 women who had a therapeutic, illegal, or spontaneous abortion, however, Wilson (1952) came to a different conclusion. He found that consequences of abortion vary with the length of the pregnancy and certain personality factors. Other studies conducted in the 1950s (Hefferman and Lynch 1953; Lidz 1954; Rosen 1958) suggested negative sequelae of abortion but many of the authors' various conclusions either were based on their own clinical opinions or appear to reflect an antiabortion bias before conducting the study.

This general opinion about the negative aftereffects of abortion persisted despite the findings from a large study (Ekblad 1955) of 479 women who had a legal abortion in Sweden. Subjects were interviewed before discharge from the hospital and 2–5 years later. Three-quarters of the women in the study did not experience regret or self-reproach after the procedure. One percent of the sample had some psychiatric problem after abortion, but all of these women had psychiatric histories. Ekblad's study was the first report that concluded there were insignificant psychiatric effects of abortion.

A study of a random sample of Swedish women evaluated 3 years after an abortion was performed found that 25% had experienced mild guilt, 23% had severe reactions, and 23% believed that their current problems were a consequence of the abortion (Aren 1958). A subsequent study of 234 Swedish women conducted 3 years after a legal abortion was performed found different results (Aren and Amark 1961). Forty-three percent of the women in the sample reported that their lives were unchanged, 37% had improved life situations, and 21% had experienced negative aftereffects.

1960–1970: Setting the Stage for Legalization of Abortion—Research Findings

The conclusion and belief that somewhat-negative psychological effects occurred after abortion (despite the methodological problems of these studies) persisted until Kummer's (1963) survey of 32 psychiatrists who frequently evaluated women after abortions. He found that 75% of the physicians had not encountered moderate or severe psychiatric reactions in patients after the procedure, whereas 25% of the respondents reported occasional negative aftereffects in their patients. The highest incidence reported was six cases in 15 years of practice. These same psychiatrists, however, reported a higher incidence of postchildbirth unfavorable psychiatric aftereffects in their patients. This study also suffered from design problems in that the investigator did not specify how the sample of psychiatrists was selected, did not specify what type of assessment methodology was used, did not specify the characteristics of the sample of patients, and failed to adjust incidence of psychiatric sequelae by incidence of abortion and live births (Shusterman 1976).

Peck and Marcus (1966) conducted a study of 50 women interviewed when they applied for an abortion and 3–6 months after the procedure.

Demographic, personal history, medical, and psychiatric data were collected in the preabortion interview. Fifty percent of the women sought an abortion for psychiatric reasons (72% were schizophrenic, 24% were depressed, and 4% were neurotic with severe character disorder); the other 50% had no psychiatric indication for the abortion. Few psychiatric effects were reported from this sample, no hospitalizations were necessary, and more of the women reported an improvement in their relationship with men. The authors concluded that abortions were therapeutic and appeared to alleviate the acute depression and anxiety resulting from having become pregnant. The onset of new psychological symptoms was mild and self-limited. This study also had methodological problems, including poor assessment measures for psychiatric outcomes and the liberal use of diagnostic labels, particularly schizophrenia, in this sample of private, nonhospitalized patients (Shusterman 1976). Similar findings were reported by Niswander and Patterson (1967), who administered a questionnaire to 116 women and found that most reported feeling improved immediately after the procedure and that this sentiment increased as time passed. Simon et al. (1967) employed objective assessment measures in addition to an interview to evaluate the effects of an abortion. They reported that psychologically healthy women, and women who had a psychiatric disorder, were generally psychologically improved after an abortion. In addition, the study reported an increase in depressive illness when an unwanted pregnancy was not terminated. Although the authors concluded that psychiatric illness sometimes occurs after abortions, the illness did not appear to be related to the procedure but rather to a preexisting psychiatric history.

Kretzschmar and Norris (1967) reported on psychiatric complications in 32 women who had therapeutic abortions during a 6-year period. These investigators found no negative psychiatric sequelae after the procedure at 1–4 years of follow-up. One methodological problem of this study was that many of the women in the sample were sterilized in addition to having received an abortion, thus making it difficult to study the effects of the abortion as an independent factor.

Additional evidence supporting the findings of mild or negligible psychological effects after abortion came from a study by Patt et al. (1969) of 35 white, young, middle-class women who were administered a semistructured interview. These authors found that the majority of women in their study reported that the abortion had positive effects with no long-term sequelae: 26 of the women found that their lives had improved over the long run, 4 had unchanged situations, and 6 felt worse. This study is complicated by its retrospective design and heavy reliance on recall data, which can be distorted with time.

The Group for the Advancement of Psychiatry (1969) reviewed the moral, ethical, psychological, and medical issues involved in abortion and supported the view that the decision for termination of pregnancy should be that of the pregnant woman. This group also recommended that before their patients undergo the procedure, physicians should explore the patients' reasons for seeking an abortion and should recommend or provide counseling when indicated. Shortly after this report was published, other mental health groups, including the American Psychiatric Association (1970) and the American Psychoanalytic Association (1970), issued reports supporting the finding of minimal psychiatric sequelae after abortion, the need for assessment and counseling procedures, and the assignment of decision making to the woman and her family.

1970–1989: Era of Legal Abortions

Marder (1970) reported on the psychological effects of the liberalization of abortion with the 1967 California Therapeutic Abortion Act, which eased access to the procedure but did not legalize it. A review of 550 cases found few serious emotional problems of guilt or remorse. Of interest was the investigator's observation that negative attitudes of hospital staff members and inadequate counseling contributed to postabortion guilt and depression.

After the law was changed to make abortion more easily available, a study from Great Britain (Pare and Raven 1970) refocused the issue on the psychological impact of bearing an unwanted child. These investigators interviewed 250 of 270 abortion seekers 1 year after a preabortion psychiatric consultation and found that all but 1 of the 128 women who had abortions were satisfied that they had terminated the pregnancy, although nearly 25% had experienced mild regret at first. The authors reported that psychiatric sequelae were more likely in overburdened multiparous women and single women who did not have adequate social supports but carried through the pregnancy. In contrast, women who had an abortion experienced few psychiatric symptoms or effects.

In one of the few prospective and methodologically sound studies of the psychological impact of therapeutic abortion, Brody et al. (1971) administered several objective assessment measures, including the Minnesota Multiphasic Personality Inventory (MMPI) to 117 applicants for abortion and to 58 "comparison" women who were in the same stage of pregnancy as those in the abortion sample. The women who received an abortion were again evaluated at 6 weeks, 6 months, and 1 year after the procedure, whereas those patients who were not granted an abortion and the comparison group were retested only 6 weeks after the initial screening. The authors concluded that the procedure is generally beneficial and effective in reducing psychopathological symptoms caused by unwanted pregnancy.

Ford et al. (1971a, 1971b, 1972) replicated the design of the Brody et al. study and demonstrated similar results. Other investigators also reported that the outcomes of therapeutic abortions were positive and that favorable consequences occurred when a woman decided that abortion was the best course of action for her (Osofsky et al. 1971; Payne et al. 1976). Osofsky and Osofsky's (1972) methodologically rigorous study of abortion on request demonstrated minimal psychiatric complications from the procedure. They interviewed 380 women (most of whom were young, white, and unmarried) immediately and 1 month after an abortion. They found that 64% of the sample felt moderately or very satisfied with the outcome of the abortion, 20% were neutral, and 15% were unhappy with the outcome. More than 75% of the sample did not experience guilt in response to the procedure and were satisfied with their decision to terminate the pregnancy. Seventy-seven percent of the sample reported wanting to have children in the future. In a follow-up article, Osofsky and Osofsky (1973) examined the psychological variables that predicted outcomes in their earlier study. They found that patients who had the greatest difficulty in their decision to seek an abortion had the most remorse and reported an enhanced desire to have future children. Moreover, this group was characterized by particular demographic characteristics, including being Catholic.

Athanasiou et al. (1973) compared psychological outcomes based on objective assessment measures of women who carried their pregnancies to term and women who received abortions. Beginning with a sample of 373 women, these investigators matched 38 women in each group for age, marital status, socioeconomic status, parity, and ethnicity. From 13 to 16 months after the abortion or the delivery, psychometric evaluations were performed including the MMPI and the Symptom Checklist 90—Revised. None of the groups exhibited psychopathology, and few differences among groups were found. The investigators concluded that there were no serious physical or psychological effects of abortion. Smith (1973) conducted a methodologically sound study of 80 young, single women, most of whom were students. He administered structured interviews 1–2 years after an abortion and found that 90% of the sample reported no negative psychological sequelae after the procedure. Furthermore, 94% were satisfied with their decision, 40% said the procedure had no impact on their lives, and an additional 40% reported that the abortion had a positive, maturing effect. Only a small minority of the sample reported any negative consequences. Two of the 15 women in the sample who had previous psychiatric histories received psychiatric interventions after the procedure. The study by Monsour and Stewart (1973) further supports these findings. These investigators studied a random sample of 20 college women who had received abortions and found predominantly positive reactions to the procedure. This study was flawed, however, by its range of follow-up times and the small size of the sample.

In a follow-up study of 126 women who received abortions for psychiatric indications, Ewing and Rouse (1973) found that the 52 women with a history of prior psychiatric illness did not experience significantly more postabortion emotional reactions than women without a psychiatric history. Ninety-six percent of the psychiatric group and 92% of the others reported that their emotional health was better or unchanged after the procedure. Partridge and colleagues (1971) followed 207 women after they had an abortion. Ninety-eight percent of the sample felt that their general health was the same or improved, and 94% felt that their mental health was the same or improved, after the procedure. Most of the emotional symptoms reported decreased over time. The authors found that a psychiatric history did not predict who would have a negative outcome after the abortion. Other investigators (Addelson 1973; Adler 1973) also found that the psychiatric results of abortion were benign.

Additional evidence for the finding that no severe psychiatric sequelae result after an abortion came from international studies (Osofsky and Osofsky 1972; Shusterman 1976). In particular, Lask (1975) found that 89% of the sample he studied had improved or unchanged psychiatric status. Although 11% had adverse reactions, their response appeared to be related more to other factors, such as a woman having a past history of psychiatric illness, ambivalence, or desertion by her partner.

One study attempted to identify predictive factors of the long-term effects of abortion. Payne et al. (1976) undertook a prospective study to identify women at risk for developing problems after abortions. These researchers studied 102 patients during four time intervals—before an abortion and in the postabortion period (24 hours, 6 weeks, and 6 months)—by using psychometric measures such as the MMPI, Profile of Mood States, symptom rating scales, and interviews. Five effects were seen as the most important dependent variables—anxiety, anger, guilt, shame, and depression. The researchers found that during the first 24 hours, women experienced great feelings of relief and a decrease in depression, guilt, and anxiety. At 6 weeks, feelings of depression, anxiety, and guilt were increased. By 6 months, however, all effects were significantly lower and returned to the baseline level. Gould (1980) suggested that women who are particularly vulnerable to postabortion depression are single and nulliparous and have a history of previous psychiatric illness, conflictual or immature relationships with lovers, past negative relationships with their mothers, negative cultural or religious views of abortions, and strong ambivalence.

Tietze (1975) found that the emotional response after an abortion paralleled psychiatric reactions seen in other crisis situations. Initially, feelings of relief predominated, and 6 months after the procedure, most women did not report sadness or depression. Those who did experience negative reactions were often single and had a previous history of psychiatric disorder; conflicted, unstable relationships with men; strong ambivalence toward the procedure; religious or cultural backgrounds that were prohibitive of abortion; and a poor relationship with their mothers. At 6-month follow-up interviews, however, these women reported that the decision to abort had been the correct course of action for them. Tietze (1975) emphasized that the presence of risk factors for psychiatric complications should not be construed as a contraindication for the procedure and that crisis-intervention techniques should be used to minimize any negative impact of the procedure.

Some studies conducted in the 1970s suggest that abortions in some women were followed by anxiety, depression, and guilt (Ford et al. 1971a, 1971b); however, a review by Illsley and Hall (1976) of many studies conducted in several countries suggests that few serious problems occur after termination of an unwanted pregnancy, although a few women will experience some adverse reaction. Brewer (1977) reported that the incidence of postabortion psychosis was .3 per 1,000 terminations compared to 1.7 per 1,000 deliveries. Belsey et al. (1977) and Greer et al. (1976) also demonstrated that adverse psychiatric reactions to abortion were rare and seemed to occur in women with prior psychiatric histories, instability, poor social supports, and preabortion ambivalence about the procedure. These studies raised the possibility that negative reactions may be a consequence of a woman's preexisting emotional difficulties and not a specific reaction to the abortion. Meikle et al. (1977), in a study comparing 100 women applying for therapeutic abortions during 1967 and 1968 with 100 applicants for the procedure in 1975, supported these findings. Results from the MMPI showed a significant decrease in psychopathology among the more recent applicants, suggesting that a more liberal social atmosphere surrounding abortion reduced the psychological sequelae and stress of the procedure. A study by Kummer and Robinson (1978) of women who had obtained an abortion issued a cautionary note, suggesting that women who had the procedure may be more vulnerable to depression and anxiety at the time of their first wanted pregnancy.

Moseley et al. (1981) investigated demographic and psychological factors in 62 women with positive or negative reactions to the procedure. They found some psychiatric aftereffects but demonstrated that the most important determinant in a woman's psychological reaction was the perceived amount of support from her significant others. Bradley (1984) evaluated 266 women in a prospective, longitudinal study to determine psychological factors associated with pregnancy and childbirth. Twenty-eight women in the sample had experienced a therapeutic abortion. The study failed to demonstrate a relationship between anxiety during pregnancy and a previous abortion, and there were no indications of inadequate maternal functioning in these women. The women who had a previous abortion had higher levels of depressive affect in the third trimester of pregnancy and in the postpartum period, but these women were not clinically depressed. Bradley concluded that there were no adverse psychological effects of a previous abortion on subsequent full-term pregnancy outcomes.

In an extensive review of the literature on the long-term psychiatric impact of abortion, Shusterman (1976) concluded that the psychiatric aftereffects of the procedure were minor and that women who choose to have abortions have no greater psychopathology than women who carry pregnancies to a full term. Walter (1970) emphasized that abortion may be more beneficial to a woman than mandatory motherhood. Lazarus (1985) supported findings from earlier research that most subjects (75%) experience relief after an abortion, followed by short-term guilt and depressive reactions in 15%. Only rare recent studies suggest possible negative outcomes. Major et al. (1985) found that among 247 women who received an abortion during the first trimester, the women who felt that their pregnancies were highly meaningful (in contrast to those who did not attach this significance to the pregnancy) experienced more negative psychological effects and had more physical complaints after the procedure. Three weeks after an abortion, women who had not wanted to be pregnant had significantly lower ratings on the Beck Depression Inventory than the women who had some desire to become pregnant. Cohen and Roth (1989) studied coping styles and levels of anxiety and depression before and immediately after an abortion. They found that women who used coping techniques demonstrated a greater decrease in anxiety from before to after an abortion than those who did not employ coping strategies. In addition, women who used denial had higher depression and anxiety scores than those who did not use this defense mechanism. Tollefson and Garvey (1983) described the development of a conversion disorder in a 25-year-old single woman as a defense mechanism against fears of pregnancy and pregnancy termination. Bradley (1984) suggested that grief, anxiety, or depression after an abortion may be unresolved and reappear in a subsequent pregnancy. There are anecdotal reports suggesting that a posttraumatic stress disorder may occur (Ney and Wickett 1989), but no systematic research has shown that this illness is a result of the procedure.

More than 200 reports on the psychological effects of abortion exist in the literature, but there are only a few well-designed studies to evaluate the consequences of the procedure (Shusterman 1976). From the research for which sound methodology was employed, the overall evidence supports the finding that therapeutic abortion and abortion on request are basically nontraumatic procedures that have minimal psychiatric complications for women.

Psychological Consequences of Denied Abortion

Few of the studies on the psychological sequelae of abortion have used a control or comparison group. In part, this is attributable to the difficulty in constructing an appropriate comparison sample. Therefore, some researchers (Nadelson and Notman 1984; Shusterman 1976) have suggested that the results of studies evaluating the psychological impact of abortion should be compared with the findings from research assessing the consequences of denied abortions.

There are numerous methodological problems with such a comparison, however. Hamill and Ingram (1974) demonstrated that women denied abortions were considered more stable by their physicians, given that a psychiatric reason was needed to obtain the procedure. Therefore, this sample of women might have constituted a different group from those who were granted the procedure. Moreover, many women who were initially refused abortions went somewhere else to undergo the procedure so that follow-up data on these women are often incomplete. Furthermore, it cannot be directly inferred that the results from this sample of women can be applied to those women who received abortions in the event the procedure had been denied (Handy 1982). Perhaps the most useful group for comparison would be women who carry to term an unwanted pregnancy and who then give the child up for adoption. This would control for both the unwantedness of the pregnancy and the experience of loss (Adler et al. 1990). Nevertheless, the studies that have been conducted do provide some useful insights.

Psychological Consequences of Illegal Abortion

The literature on illegal abortion, albeit dated, provides an interesting comparison to the research on therapeutic abortion. An illegal abortion is extremely different from the therapeutic procedure. Illegal abortions tend to be clandestine, expensive, and performed by individuals who are not fully competent. Shusterman (1976) emphasized that there are considerable methodological problems in trying to study something that is illegal, including the lack of standardization of the quality of the procedure, the practitioner's experience, and the accuracy of the information provided. The process of obtaining the abortion is often dangerous and humiliating, and there is a higher incidence of medical complications (Lee 1969; Schulder and Kennedy 1971). Nonetheless, Lee (1969) found that only 8% of women who received an illegal abortion had severe emotional problems and fewer than 50% were depressed after the procedure. Negative psychological effects seemed to disappear after several weeks.

Psychological Consequences of Carrying Through
an Unintended Pregnancy

Caplan (1954) found disturbed relationships between mothers and children when abortions had been denied during pregnancy. In a study of 213 children born to women who had been refused therapeutic abortions, Hook

(1963) found that unwanted children had greater physical and emotional disabilities than control subjects. In an important study, Forssman and Thuwe (1966) followed—for 21 years—120 Swedish children who were born after an application for a therapeutic abortion was denied. These children were compared with matched control subjects of same-sex children born on the same day in the same district of the country. The initial results indicated that the unwanted children had poorer outcomes in almost every way, including higher incidences of psychiatric disorders, alcoholism, delinquency, and criminal behavior. They were more often receiving public assistance, received less education, and were often exempted from military service for medical or psychiatric reasons. The researchers concluded that the psychological and social consequences of denied abortions were often more serious than those associated with abortion. They hypothesized that pregnancy might bring punitive consequences to a woman if the child was illegitimate, with subsequent feelings of resentment toward the unborn child (Handy 1982). Carrying through an unwanted pregnancy results in years of responsibility for a child, often under adverse circumstances, and this (in contrast to a terminated pregnancy) may produce lasting stress and psychiatric problems for both mother and child (Handy 1982). Forssman and Thuwe (1966) concluded that children born after unwanted pregnancies had greater social and psychological impairment than their peers and recommended that these factors be weighed when evaluating reasons for recommending therapeutic abortions. A follow-up report by Forssman and Thuwe (1981), after 31 years of studying this cohort, revealed that the index cases as a group had poorer social and psychiatric outcomes than the control subjects; however, the initial pronounced differences between the two groups found in earlier studies had leveled out somewhat.

Other studies confirm these findings of negative psychological sequelae resulting from an unwanted pregnancy. Pare and Raven (1970) found that at 1-year follow-up, one-third of women denied an abortion regretted this outcome and resented the baby. Visram (1971) reported similar adverse outcomes: More than one-third of the 95 women denied abortions had not coped with their situation, 6 had made suicide attempts, 2 had committed suicide, and more than 50% of the children were being raised in adverse circumstances. Zabin et al. (1989) interviewed 360 adolescents who received pregnancy tests and compared the young women who had negative results with those who were pregnant and carried to term and with those who received abortions. All three groups demonstrated higher levels of transient anxiety at the baseline level compared with follow-up 1–2 years later. Two years after the procedure, the abortion group exhibited a more positive psychological profile than the other two groups. The abortion group had lower levels of trait anxiety than either of the other groups and demonstrated greater self-esteem than the negative-pregnancy group and a greater sense of internal control than the childbearing group. Subsequent studies by other investigators of risk factors for child abuse and neglect repeat these authors' warnings about the fate and negative outcomes of unwanted children (Handy 1982; Kempe 1976; Prescott 1976; Resnick 1969).

Conclusions

The pendulum of thought concerning the psychiatric impact of abortion has swung 180 degrees during the past 40 years (Friedman et al. 1974). The literature of the 1940s and 1950s reported on the presumed traumatic effects of the procedure, despite the lack of substantiative findings to support this conclusion (Friedman et al. 1974). In the 1960s and 1970s, the literature focused on the minimal psychological effects of abortion, and what effects were reported appeared to decrease as time passed. Several studies suggested that an abortion may have some positive effects, such as contributing to a young woman's emotional maturation and growth (Notman et al. 1972). The few studies conducted in the 1980s confirm the reports of the previous two decades that there are few psychiatric sequelae of the procedure. Yet this decade has also brought a resurgence of clinical anecdotes about negative aftereffects of the procedure. The 1989 Surgeon General's Report reviewed the scientific literature on the public health effects of abortion and, although concluding that negative aftereffects were rare, stressed the inadequacy of research on the procedure, recommending prospective, longitudinal research on the physical health and mental health effects of reproductive events in general.

Since the 1973 Supreme Court decision to eliminate the need for a therapeutic indication to obtain an abortion, women have had access to the procedure with minimal medical or psychiatric risks. The increasing availability and utilization of legal abortion in the United States had several public health effects in the 1970s and 1980s, including reduction in deaths and surgical complications among women of childbearing age, the development of safer surgical procedures for pregnancy termination, and the increased provision of low-cost outpatient gynecological services (Cates 1982). During the past decade, replacement of unintended births and illegal abortions has averted perhaps 2,000 pregnancy-related deaths and several tens of thousands of life-threatening complications (Tietze 1984). Nevertheless, the *Webster v. Reproductive Health Services* (1989) decision and other pending Supreme Court cases once again raise the specter of restricted access to the procedure, which may in turn have potentially serious implications and consequences for women's mental and physical health.

Research on the psychological impact of abortion has focused on outcomes after illegal abortion, therapeutic abortion, and abortions that are requested. The studies of the first two types have generally been methodologically flawed and lacked standardized objective measurements, comparison groups, or statistical analyses. They are also often retrospective in nature, further complicating interpretation of the conclusions (Shusterman 1976). Research that has examined abortions on request has generally been methodologically sound; therefore, greater validity can be given to the conclusions drawn from these studies. This research has demonstrated that the abortion population tends to be young, single women who are not prepared or willing to change their lives to have a child because of social, occupational, and financial constraints (Shusterman 1976).

Despite methodological problems encountered in any one study, the preponderance of scientific literature on legalized abortion with diverse samples, different psychometric measures, and different kinds of assessment suggests that for most women, abortion is accompanied by emotional relief from what would be more stressful life events, an unwanted pregnancy, or an illegal abortion. The time of greatest distress is most often before the procedure. Although short-term grief, guilt, and depressive reactions may occur in relation to an abortion, long-term psychiatric sequelae are rare. The proportion of women with serious aftereffects is between 5% and 10%, and differential reactions may occur among various ethnic and cultural groups. These severe reactions can best be understood in the context of coping with a stressful life event. Former Surgeon General Koop testified before the U.S. Congress regarding his review of the scientific literature on the psychological effects of abortion. He acknowledged that responses to an abortion can be overwhelming for a particular woman, but he indicated that the development of significant problems is "minuscule from a public health perspective" (Surgeon General's Report 1989). The dearth of literature studying the delayed consequences of undesired pregnancy and abortion or having an unwanted child raises some unanswered questions. How do events linked by reproduction, such as an abortion or carrying to term an unwanted pregnancy—experiences that involve both psychological and biological stressors—relate to increasing vulnerability for affective disorders or other psychiatric illnesses during the lives of women? For many women, these pregnancy-related events occur during their teens and twenties when women are at increased risk for the development of mood disorders. Does an abortion or an unwanted pregnancy represent a psychobiological event that may sensitize or trigger the development of affective syndromes later in life? What are the relationships between abortion or unwanted pregnancy and reproduction-related affective syndromes, such as postpartum depressive illness? Are there associations between these events and the development of an anxiety disorder, particularly posttraumatic stress disorder? Conversely, does an abortion protect a woman from the potentially greater psychological and biological stress and anxiety of carrying to term an unwanted pregnancy? To what extent do personality traits and disorders and sociodemographic factors influence abortion outcomes?

There is no scientific literature supporting the relationship of having an abortion to the subsequent development of an affective or anxiety disorder, and the questions in the previous paragraph are purely speculative. The research literature does not show an increased risk for affective illness or anxiety disorders in women who have had abortions, but it does demonstrate that unwanted pregnancy carries with it an increased risk for psychiatric disorder. What are the risk factors for negative psychological reactions, and how can knowledge of these variables be translated into effective intervention strategies? Further basic and clinical studies in these areas are needed. Applying new research advances in psychiatric assessment methodology to these questions should enhance our ability to predict who is at risk for the development of psychiatric problems and whether difficulties after an abortion may relate to a previous history of psychiatric disorder.

Longitudinal, prospective research is needed to answer these questions, to assess the incidence and prevalence of psychological outcomes of reproductive events during the life cycle (including menarche, pregnancy, abortion, the postpartum period, and menopause), and to determine what antecedent psychological variables may contribute to these outcomes. Furthermore, research is urgently needed on methods to change high-risk sexual behavior to prevent unwanted pregnancy. Not enough is known about why sexually active men and women are willing to risk unintended pregnancy when safe and effective family planning is available. We need to understand better the causes and correlates of risk-taking behavior and develop strategies for the translation of knowledge about how to prevent unwanted pregnancy into effective and consistent contraceptive practices (Surgeon General's Report 1989).

Despite being a safe procedure under proper professional medical supervision, an abortion carries a particular emotional significance for an individual woman, given that it represents the termination of a pregnancy. Such a decision is always painful and difficult, should be considered carefully, and should be weighed against the benefits and costs of carrying the pregnancy to term. In this regard, various options need to be developed for women, with adequate resources committed to support them. According to Koop (Surgeon General's Report 1989),

> if our society wants fewer abortions, it must be willing to support not only those children who are so born, but also the women who make that choice. As a society, we must make a commitment to provide loving families for all children placed for adoption. When women decide to bear their own children, rather than stigmatize them, we must sustain them by ensuring subsidized prenatal and delivery costs, foster care, day care benefits for the working mother and educational and job guarantees during maternity leave. The sexual partners of such women should be held jointly responsible for the mother and child's medical cost and for child support. (p. 23)

Since these kinds of societal measures are still far in the future, however, abortion remains a necessary option for many women lacking the emotional, financial, or social resources necessary to carry through a pregnancy. Similarly, it represents an option of choice for those women who do not want (for various reasons) to carry through an unwanted pregnancy. Thus, it is crucial that we invest in prevention, because "every abortion represents a failure of both the individual and of the society to apply knowledge about contraception into effective and consistent practices" (Surgeon General's Report 1989). It is these failures of prevention that result in the needless personal crises that an abortion decision represents for women, their sexual partners, and their families.

The importance of counseling in decisions about abortion must be stressed. Information about various options available to women—including abortion, adoption, and choosing to raise a child—should be presented in an unbiased manner. Preabortion and postabortion counseling, careful psychiatric and medical history taking, and the provision of support—delivered in the context of respect for the woman's individual decision making and control over her own future—should further minimize any negative consequences of the procedure.

References

Addelson F: Induced abortion: source of guilt or growth? Am J Orthopsychiatry 43:815–823, 1973

Adler N: Dimensions underlying emotional responses of women following therapeutic abortion. Paper presented at the annual meeting of the American Psychological Association, Montreal, August 1973

Adler N, David H, Major B, et al: Psychological responses after abortion. Science 248:41–43, 1990

American Psychiatric Association: Position statement on abortion. Am J Psychiatry 126:1554, 1970

American Psychiatric Association: Diagnostic and Statistical Manual of Mental Disorders, 3rd Edition, Revised. Washington, DC, American Psychiatric Association, 1987

American Psychoanalytic Association: Position statement on abortion. San Francisco, CA, American Psychoanalytic Association, 1970

Aren P: Legal abortion in Sweden. Acta Obstet Gynecol Scand Suppl 36, 1958

Aren P, Amark C: The prognosis in cases in which legal abortion has been granted but not carried out. Acta Obstet Gynecol Scand 36:203–278, 1961

Athanasiou R, Michelson L, Oppel W, et al: Psychiatric sequelae to term birth and induced early and late abortion: a longitudinal study. Fam Plann Perspect 5:227–231, 1973

Belsey EM, Greer HS, Lai S, et al: Predictive factors in response to abortion: King's Termination Study IV. Soc Sci Med 2:71–82, 1977

Bradley CF: Abortion and subsequent pregnancy. Can J Psychiatry 29:494–498, 1984

Brewer C: Incidence of post-abortion psychosis: a prospective study. Br Med J 1:476–477, 1977

Brody H, Meikle S, Gerritse R: Therapeutic abortion: a prospective study. Am J Obstet Gynecol 109:347–352, 1971

Caplan G: The disturbance of the mother-child relationship by unsuccessful attempts at abortion. Mental Hygiene 38:67–80, 1954

Cates WC: Legal abortion: the public health record. Science 215:1586–1590, 1982

Cohen L, Roth S: Coping with abortion. Journal of Human Stress 10:140–145, 1989

David HP, Rasmussen NK, Holst E: Postpartum and post abortion psychotic reactions. Fam Plann Perspect 13:88–92, 1981

Doane BK, Quigley BG: Psychiatric aspects of therapeutic abortion. CMA Journal 125:427–432, 1981

Doe v. Bolton, 410 U.S. 179 (1973)

Ebaugh F, Hesuer A: Psychiatric aspects of therapeutic abortion. Postgrad Med 2:325–332, 1947

Ekblad N: Induced abortion on psychiatric grounds. Acta Psychiatr Neurol Scand Suppl 99:1–238, 1955

Ewing JW, Rouse BA: Therapeutic abortion and a prior psychiatric history. Am J Psychiatry 130:37–40, 1973

Ford C, Atkinson R, Bragonier J: Therapeutic abortion: who needs a psychiatrist? Obstet Gynecol 38:206–213, 1971a

Ford C, Castelnuova-Tedesco P, Long K: Is abortion a therapeutic procedure in psychiatry? JAMA 218:1173–1178, 1971b

Ford C, Castelnuova-Tedesco P, Long K: Women who seek abortion: a comparison with women who complete their pregnancies. Am J Psychiatry 129:546–552, 1972

Forssman H, Thuwe I: One hundred and twenty children born after application for therapeutic abortion was refused: their mental health, social adjustment and educational level up to the age of 21. Acta Psychiatr Scand 42:71–88, 1966

Forssman H, Thuwe I: Continued follow-up study of 120 persons born after refusal of application for therapeutic abortion. Acta Psychiatr Scand 64:142–149, 1981

Friedman CM, Greenspan R, Mittleman F: The decision-making process and outcome of therapeutic abortion. Am J Psychiatry 131:1332–1336, 1974

Gould NB: Postabortion depressive reactions in college women. J Am Coll Health Assoc 28:316–320, 1980

Greer HS, Lai S, Lewis SC, et al: Psychological consequences of therapeutic abortion: King's Termination Study III. Br J Psychiatry 128:74–79, 1976

Group for the Advancement of Psychiatry: The Right to Abortion: A Psychiatric View. New York, Group for the Advancement of Psychiatry, 1969

Hamill E, Ingram IM: Psychiatric and social factors in the abortion decision. Br Med J 1:229–232, 1974

Hamilton V: Some sociologic and psychologic observations on abortion. Am J Obstet Gynecol 39:919–928, 1940

Hamilton V: Medical status and psychologic attitudes of patients following abortion. Am J Obstet Gynecol 41:285–287, 1941

Handy JA: Psychological and social aspects of induced abortion. Br J Clin Psychol 21:29–41, 1982

Hefferman R, Lynch W: What is the status of therapeutic abortion in modern obstetrics? Am J Obstet Gynecol 66:335–345, 1953

Henshaw SK: Induced abortion: a worldwide perspective. Fam Plann Perspect 18:250–255, 1986

Hesseltine H, Adair F, Boynton M: Limitation of human reproduction: therapeutic abortion. Am J Obstet Gynecol 39:549–562, 1940

Hook K: Refused abortion: a follow-up of 249 women whose applications were refused by the National Board of Health in Sweden. Acta Psychiatr Scand Suppl 168:39, 1963

Illsley R, Hall MH: Psychosocial aspects of abortion. Bull WORLD Health Organ 52:83–106, 1976

Kempe C: Approaches to preventing child abuse: a health visitor's concept. Am J Dis Child 130:941, 1976

Kretzschmar R, Norris A: Psychiatric implications of therapeutic abortion. Am J Obstet Gynecol 198:368–373, 1967

Kummer J: Post abortion psychiatric illness—a myth? Am J Psychiatry 119:980–983, 1963

Kummer J, Robinson K: Previous induced abortion and ante-natal depression in primiparae: preliminary report of a survey of mental health in pregnancy. Psychol Med 8:711–715, 1978

Lask B: Short-term psychiatric sequelae to therapeutic termination of pregnancy. Br J Psychiatry 126:173–177, 1975

Lazarus A: Psychiatric sequelae of legalized elective first trimester abortion. Journal of Psychosomatic Obstetrics and Gynecology 4:141–150, 1985

Lee N: The Search for an Abortionist. Chicago, IL, University of Chicago Press, 1969

Lidz T: Reflections of a psychiatrist, in Therapeutic Abortion. Edited by Rosen H. New York, Julian Press, 1954, pp 276–283

Major B, Mueller P, Hildebrandt K: Attributions, expectations, and coping with abortion. J Pers Soc Psychol 48:585–599, 1985

Marder L: Psychiatric experience with a liberalized therapeutic abortion law. Am J Psychiatry 126:1230–1236, 1970

Meikle S, Robinson C, Brody H: Recent changes in the emotional reactions of therapeutic abortion applicants. Can Psychiatr Assoc J 22:67–70, 1977

Monsour K, Stewart B: Abortion and sexual behavior in college women. Am J Orthopsychiatry 43:804–813, 1973

Moseley DT, Follingstad DR, Harley H: Psychological factors that predict reaction to abortion. J Clin Psychol 37:276–279, 1981

Nadelson C: Psychological issues in therapeutic abortion. J Am Med Wom Assoc 27:12–15, 1972

Nadelson CC, Notman MT: The emotional impact of abortion, in The Woman Patient, Vol 1: Sexual and Reproductive Aspects of Women's Health Care. Edited by Notman MT, Nadelson CC. New York, Preliminary Press, 1984, pp 173–179

Ney PG, Wickett AR: Mental health and abortion: review and analysis. Psychiatr J Univ Ottawa 14:506–516, 1989

Niswander K, Patterson R: Psychologic reaction to therapeutic abortion. Obstet Gynecol 29:702–706, 1967

Notman M, Kravitz A, Payne E, et al: Psychological outcome in patients having therapeutic abortions, in Psychosomatic Medicine in Obstetrics and Gynecology: Third International Congress. Edited by Morris T. Basel, Karger, 1972, pp 552–554

Osofsky JD, Osofsky HJ: The psychological reaction of patients to legalized abortion. Am J Orthopsychiatry 42:48–60, 1972

Osofsky JD, Osofsky HJ: The Abortion Experience: Psychological and Medical Impact. Hagerstown, MD, Harper & Row, 1973

Osofsky J, Osofsky H, Rajan R: Psychological effects of legal abortion. Clin Obstet Gynecol 14:215–234, 1971

Pare C, Raven H: Follow-up of patients referred for termination of pregnancy. Lancet 1:635–638, 1970

Partridge J, Spiegel T, Rouse B, et al: Therapeutic abortion: a study of psychiatric applicants at North Carolina Memorial Hospital. N C Med J 32:132–136, 1971

Pasnau R: Psychiatric complications of therapeutic abortion. Obstet Gynecol 40:252–256, 1972

Patt S, Rappaport R, Barglow P: Follow-up of therapeutic abortion. Arch Gen Psychiatry 20:408–414, 1969

Payne E, Kravitz A, Notman M, et al: Outcome following therapeutic abortion. Arch Gen Psychiatry 33:725–733, 1976

Peck A, Marcus H: Psychiatric sequelae of therapeutic interruption of pregnancy. J Nerv Ment Dis 143:417–425, 1966

Prescott JW: Abortion or the unwanted child: a choice for a humanistic society. J Pediatr Psychol 1:62–67, 1976

Resnick P: Child murder by parents: a psychiatric review of filicide. Am J Psychiatry 126:325–334, 1969

Roe v. Wade, 410 U.S. 113 (1973)

Rosen H: Other aspects of the abortion problem, in Abortion in the United States. Edited by Calderone M. New York, Hoeber & Harper, 1958, pp 129–131

Schulder D, Kennedy F: Abortion Rap. New York, McGraw-Hill, 1971

Shusterman LR: The psychosocial factors of the abortion experience: a critical review. Psychology of Women Quarterly 1:79–106, 1976

Simon N, Senturia A, Rothman D: Psychiatric illness following therapeutic abortion. Am J Psychiatry 126:1224–1229, 1967

Smith E: A follow-up study of women who request abortion. Am J Orthopsychiatry 43:574–585, 1973

Surgeon General's Report on the Public Health Effects of Abortion. Unpublished document. Washington, DC, 1989

Tietze C: Contraceptive practice in the context of a non-restrictive abortion law. Fam Plann Perspect 7:197–202, 1975

Tietze C: The public health effects of legal abortion in the United States. Fam Plann Perspect 16:26–28, 1984

Tollefson GD, Garvey MJ: Conversion disorder following termination of pregnancy. J Fam Pract 16:73–77, 1983

Visram SA: A follow-up study of 95 women who were refused abortion on psychiatric grounds, in Proceedings of the Third International Congress of Psychosomatic Medicine in Obstetrics and Gynecology. Edited by Morris N. Basel, Karger, 1971

Walter G: Psychologic and emotional consequences of elective abortion. Obstet Gynecol 36:482–487, 1970

Webster v. Reproductive Health Services, 109 S.Ct. 3040 (1989)

Whittington H: Evaluation of therapeutic abortion as an element of preventive psychiatry. Am J Psychiatry 126:1224–1229, 1970

Wilson D: Psychiatric indications for abortion. Virginia Medical Monthly 79:448–451, 1952

Wilson D, Caine B: The psychiatric implications of therapeutic abortions. Neuropsychiatry 1:22, 1951

Zabin LS, Hirsch MB, Emerson MR: When urban adolescents choose abortion: effects on education, psychological status and subsequent pregnancy. Fam Plann Perspect 21:248–255, 1989

Chapter 3

Historical and Cross-Cultural Perspectives on Abortion

Lucile F. Newman, Ph.D.

A ll humans have experienced curiosity about what human life is. What is the nature of aliveness? Who are we? How are we defined as people? Many societies maintain a belief in the conservation of the soul in a cycle of life, death, and rebirth. Others believe that the first objective of life is to achieve oblivion, that the soul of an individual is consigned at birth to a heaven or hell, or that death is the end of existence for the individual while continuity inheres in the conservation of matter or cell life. How, then, can life be defined?

Through history and among cultures, certain variations occur in the definition of life—whether it is potentiality, motion, consciousness, or insight or whether it inheres in individual existence or social recognition. The various definitions of life indicate that the beginning of life, rather than a biological point where life is infused, has a cultural definition depending on a people's beliefs about a soul, reincarnation, social structure, kinship, and community and other surrounding beliefs. In this chapter, I address abortion through the perspective of biological quality control, through some historical perspectives on the definition of life, through cross-cultural views of the social control of reproduction, and through the perspective of the human costs of unwantedness.

Biological Quality Control

In the process of human embryonic and fetal development, there is loss at every level. Embryonic loss in the first weeks after conception has been estimated at 50–78% (Roberts and Lowe 1975; Shepard and Fantel 1979). Many of these losses are results of genetic configurations inconsistent with life, such as trisomy 16, or occur because of incompatibility of the embryonic organism and maternal environment. Others are of unknown origin. Such losses may be experienced as a late or missed menstrual period, or they may not be noticed at all. Roberts and Lowe (1975) and Shepard and Fantel (1979) suggested that the elimination of genetically malformed or mismatched embryos may be an important contribution to human reproductive success. Although malformation seems to be the norm rather than the exception in the development of early embryos, mechanisms that reject more than half of conceptive organisms work toward a kind of biological quality control on the human species (Roberts and Lowe 1975; Wasser 1990). Shepard and Fantel (1979) suggested that the most severe of these genetic anomalies are ended earliest.

A second level of loss results from a failure to implant—perhaps because of an inhospitable uterine environment, uterine disease, or misplacement of the embryonic fetal organism (as in ectopic pregnancy). Postimplantation fetal loss may be caused by maternal trauma, exposure to or ingestion of toxic substances, blood or biochemical incompatibility, or individual or unknown causes. Some losses during this period result from deliberate action to provoke abortion. Therapeutic abortion may be used to avoid having a child with a known abnormality, such as a neural tube defect, or a known disease incompatible with normal life, such as Tay-Sachs disease.

From week 20 to week 24, with an established pregnancy and perceived fetal movement, there is less loss experienced; however, some later spontaneous abortions occur at all levels until the point of individual viability. After that time, fetuses appear as preterm births. With the current scientific apparatus of neonatal intensive care, viability occurs at about 6 months (24–26 weeks gestation). Some slightly smaller infants born at 23 weeks are kept alive for some time although with difficult outcomes and variable prognoses. Although the point of viability had been occurring earlier during pregnancy in the past decade, 24–25 weeks appears to be the earliest point of viability, at which perhaps half of all fetuses will be able to live normal lives.

Evidence from in vitro fertilization research has contributed to our understanding of the extent of embryonic loss from individual genetic defects and from incompatible gametes. Knowledge that every conception does not hold or does not lead to a pregnancy and that a pregnancy does not necessarily lead to a viable birth provides the first context for thinking about abortion, since natural forms of biological control are already in force. Interest in the social circumstances of birth, the quality of life, and avoidance of unwanted children provides a second context of social concern. These concerns have been expressed throughout history in varying definitions of life.

Historical Perspectives on the Definition of Life

The definition of human life has been a matter of tradition and convention in every society throughout history. Reflections on what constitutes the beginning of a human life indicate the cultural nature of this issue. The geneticist Joshua Lederberg, in suggesting a continuum of life, pointed out that scientific observation shows development to be a gradual elaboration of the potentialities inherent in every cell (Lederberg 1966, p. 521). That is, there is no physiological infusion of life at a given point. There is only growth and differentiation. In no society is there a sense of loss at the monthly passing of an ovum or at the flushing away of 100,000 sperm, all of which carry DNA and the potential for human life. Fertilization initiates a process of cell division, but, as I noted before, only about half of the fertilized ova result in a pregnancy. The cultural decision about when a growing, developing, and adapting organism should be endowed with human rights is based on custom, not biology.

People in every society have had specific views on the beginning of human life. The Hippocratic authors of the fifth century B.C. postulated that humanity was accomplished at 30 days gestation for a male and 42 days for a female. Aristotle agreed on the earlier animation of the male embryo, but he put the times at 40 and 90 days, respectively. He concluded that that which was alive had soul in it, itself indicated by movement and sensation (McKeon 1941). Galen, reverting to the ancient value of the quarantine (40-day period) as a special time period in human life, established the 40th day for both male and female, a decision accepted by Roman civil law. Later, English common law defined life as beginning at the time of quickening, an archaic term denoting the time, at about the 5th month of gestation, when a fetus is felt to move. Thomas Aquinas defined the soul as the first principle of life and life as signalized by two factors—knowledge and movement. Although the soul and knowledge of the unborn were not manifest, movement at about 5 months of gestation was unmistakable, and Aquinas, too, postulated quickening as the point of animation and the beginning of a particular human life (Newman 1967).

In some Polynesian societies, life has been perceived to begin with the first breath, when an infant "inhales a soul." In others, humanity is not established until after an infant's first cry or after the infant is named a member of a clan. In villages of India, the 10th-day ceremony when the infant is named traditionally marks the beginning of life (Karve 1965).

These definitions of life all have one thing in common. There is no social recognition if growth ends before the culturally defined point at which the human life is said to commence. That is, no ritual or ceremony is held. In Indian villages, if an infant dies before the 10th-day ceremony, it is buried as one would bury a placenta, rather than cremated as a human being. In the United States and much of western Europe, a fetal death is marked by no public ceremonial recognition. Some of these variations represent differing philosophical concepts of humanness and animation. Other, postbirth, definitions of life have occurred in areas of high infant mortality and may reflect a protective need not to define a fetus as alive until it is clearly viable.

These examples have focused on the definition of life and indicate the broad range of such definitions. Although definitions of life may reflect specific elements of philosophy, they may be seen as protection against natural fetal loss or infant mortality.

Less specific definitions characterize the modern world with its understanding of the complexity of human development. Luker (1984) pointed out that one common area of concern for pro-life and pro-choice women activists is the use of multiple abortions rather than available contraception for fertility regulation. The opposition of pro-life women is understandable in that they oppose any abortion. The concern of pro-choice women reflects a gradualist view of developing personhood: "A fetus may not be fully a person until it is viable, but it does have potential rights at all times, and these rights increase in moral weight as the pregnancy continues" (Luker 1984, p. 108). The perception, then, is of prenatal human development ranging from ovum to viable individual, differently definable at each stage of pregnancy. This is reflected in numerous national laws that allow open abortion options in the first trimester of pregnancy and impose some restrictions on the later weeks of gestation. This gradualist view is expressed explicitly in the U.S. Supreme Court *Roe v. Wade* (1973) decision as separation of the first trimester when abortion is accepted, to the third trimester as it approaches viability, when there is perceived a "compelling state interest" in the developing fetal existence. The intervening trimester is, in the document containing the decision, reserved to individual-state decision.

International laws reflect some gradualist views of developing personhood as well as increasing consciousness of the family and social situation of women seeking abortions. In the past decade, 35 nations have enacted liberalized abortion laws, whereas the grounds for abortion have been limited in Israel, Honduras, and Romania (Cook and Dickens 1988). Some of the liberalized laws have added early (adolescent) and late maternal age pregnancy, acquired immunodeficiency syndrome or human immunodeficiency virus infection, and inadequate family circumstances as indications for permissible abortions. Some countries have removed abortion from the realm of criminal law and moved it to the realm of medical procedure. Among legislative decriminalization actions based on inadequate family circumstances, Italy, Cyprus, and Taiwan have established a woman's family welfare as grounds for abortion; France and the Netherlands have enabled abortion in situations of a woman's distress. Hungary has specified pregnancy of unwed women, separation from partner, and inadequate housing as grounds for abortion (Cook and Dickens 1988; Elias and Annas 1987).

Judicial changes toward decriminalization have occurred in Canada, where an existing prohibition of abortion was held unconstitutional for violating the integrity and security of women. In addition, England, France, Israel, the United States, and Yugoslavia have refused to allow a male veto of an abortion even when paternity is not in doubt.

In terms of definitions of life, international legislative and judicial approaches have not defined when conception occurs or when viability might begin. Numerous countries, including Austria, West Germany, Liberia, New Zealand, and the Netherlands, have reserved abortion-law action until after implantation of a fertilized ovum. Given the high rate of embryonic loss, this obviates the necessity of establishing whether there was, in fact, a pregnancy until implantation and participation in the maternal placental system is established.

Folk beliefs have some similar concerns. The indeterminacy of when conception takes place for each woman is reflected in other cultural practices, including menstrual regulation by taking specified herbal infusions or certain over-the-counter drugs to "bring on the period." Under these circumstances, a late period is perceived as unhealthy, a blockage to be relieved by these actions (Basker 1986; Newman 1965, 1972, 1980, 1985). Belief systems in Islamic societies, such as Bangladesh, may oppose abortion but not oppose menstrual regulation on the basis that it occurs before there can be a valid pregnancy test and therefore cannot be construed as the abortion of a pregnancy. Some physicians interpret the Koran as allowing abortion until 16 weeks into a pregnancy (Akhter and Rider 1983; Rosenberg et al. 1981).

Ngin (1985) described folk beliefs of two Chinese communities in Malaysia that include a perception of the embryo as a clot of blood until after the second missed period. Over-the-counter herbal clot-dispersing medicines may then be used to accomplish menstrual regulation.

Other belief systems, particularly those whose cosmology includes a belief in reincarnation, may oppose abortion. For the Hmong of inland Laos and Thailand, the souls of the dead are thought to await rebirth into their own clan. Therefore, tampering with the reproductive system would deny a clansman the rebirth assured by virtue of clan membership (Symonds 1988). All of these beliefs have an inner logic based on certain perceptions of the outer world beyond reproduction itself but of which reproduction is a part.

Cross-Cultural Perspectives on Social Control of Reproduction

Another form of definition and control occurs with strict marriage rules: Who may and may not marry? What is considered a family? Who may be a member of the clan or kinship group? Sex and social continuity have been of profound concern in all societies. They have appeared as an aspect of the ancient and universal desire to regulate membership in society and the behavior of individual members. Therefore, membership in society is defined and protected by rules for mate selection, sexual behavior, and continuity. Reproductive decisions, then, are socialized decisions—choices among alternatives politically, socially, and traditionally limited. Fertility that does not conform to the rules for membership in society has been subject to rejection. There is no biological correlate to the concept of the misbegotten, which refers to inappropriateness of parentage, pregnancy, number, spacing, timing, or location of childbearing. Membership in society may be denied to those born out of wedlock, to twins, or to those born far from home (Newman 1985, p. 3).

Throughout history there have been many variations on the subject of birth and acceptance into society. In the Roman era, 1,900 years ago, the birth of a child was not an assurance of citizenship. Infants of free citizens were received into society only as the paterfamilias willed. Contraception, abortion, exposure, and infanticide were common and not illegal practices (Dickison 1973; Feen 1983; Golden 1981; Veyne 1987, p. 9). Fourteen percent of the medicinal herbs in the "Herbal" of Dioscorides, first written at the same time, were "emmenagogues," substances taken to "bring on the period" of women who did not wish to bear a child at that time. Many others were designated as contraceptives. When these methods were not effective, a problematic birth might occur. A child whose father did not wish to raise him or her was exposed at a distance from the house or in a public place where he or she might be found and raised by someone else, often a person who would raise the child as a slave. Historical sources in large part agree that the fate of such infants would often be to grow up as slaves (Boswell 1988; Brunt 1971; Fuchs 1984). Malformed infants were exposed or drowned. This, said Seneca, was not wrath but reason: "What is good must be set apart from that which is good for nothing" (Veyne 1987, p. 10).

As the Christian church began to seek control of marriage and family life, it also attempted to control the abandonment of infants to possibly non-Christian lives. During the Middle Ages, infants were taken and given as "oblation" to a monastery, to belong thereafter to the church. Later, churches established hospices for the placement of abandoned children. The first known effort was that of Frere Guy, at Montpelier in 1180, who established the first hospice or shelter for sick or abandoned children. Infants would be left anonymously in the window grate (later to be developed into a kind of revolving cradle called a *tour*, or tower). This maintained the mother's anonymity and assured the child sustenance and work. The fate of these infants, sent out to wet nurses for the first 3 years, was to live in the hospice and then to be apprenticed out to learn a skill or trade at about age 7. Fuchs (1984, p. 2) noted that "church officials accepted the ease and secrecy of abandonment as an alternative to infanticide; conversely, state officials sought to discover and record the name and civil status of the mother and make abrogation of parental responsibility more difficult. The *tour* thus came to represent easy abandonment and became a focus of conflict between church and state in the nineteenth century."

By the 1700s, the major cities of France and Italy were recording baptisms and the number of infants kept at the hospices, indicating a rate of abandonment of children ranging from about 10% at the beginning of the century to 30–40% at the end of the century, including the cities of Paris, Toulouse, Lyons, Florence, and Milan (Boswell 1988, p. 15).

These indications of unwantedness, whether informal or served by the church, have been consistent features of social life since the beginning of recorded time. Indeed, they still exist. Some modern states, whether under religious control or for other reasons, prohibit contraception and abortion, resulting in enforced childbearing and numerous individuals without a stake in society (Osofsky 1973). In some of their cities, abandoned and unwanted children roam the streets, commit crimes, sell drugs, and create a shadow economy outside the law.

Unwantedness

Involuntary childbearing creates human costs as well as monetary and social costs. The world laboratory of nations with differing rules and customs has enabled the comparative study of the results of unwanted pregnancy. Evidence about unwantedness appears in many studies, both longitudinal and cross-sectional. All indicate learning and health deficiencies in children who were unwanted at birth. These studies were compiled and described by David et al. (1988).

The first of these studies is of the Göteborg cohort from 1939 to 1977 (Forssman and Thuwe 1981). Abortion was legalized in Sweden in 1939 under specific indications, including danger to the life of the mother, age younger than 15, and pregnancy resulting from rape, incest, or exploitation or under circumstances of mental illness or potentially inherited disease. This study is about 120 children born to women who were refused abortion (unwanted pregnancy, UP) and 120 control children, the next same-sex infants born in the same hospital, whose mothers had not sought abortion (accepted pregnancy, AP). Their compared situations included 32 (26.7%) of the unwanted pregnancies and 9 (7.5%) of the accepted pregnancies out of wedlock. Eight of the UP children were adopted and reared by other parents. None of the AP children was adopted.

The main study, which took place when the children were age 15, was based on a follow-up review of official records of the institutions of Göteborg. Findings included reports to children's aid bureaus about unsatisfactory conditions at home (17 UP, 6 AP), removal of a child from home (2 UP, 0 AP), placement in a foster home (19 UP, 4 AP), placement in a children's home (30 UP, 10 AP), and parents divorced before a child was 15 (23 UP, 13 AP). The authors concluded that the UP children were at greater risk for insecurity in childhood than the AP children.

At age 21, significant differences included those coming to psychiatric attention (28.3% UP, 15% AP), registration for delinquency (18.3% UP, 8.3% AP), and those receiving some form of public assistance between the ages of 16 and 21 (14.2% UP, 2.5% AP). In terms of educational achievement, 14.2% of the UP group had received some form of secondary-school education compared to 33.3% of the AP control subjects. Among the 77 pairs matched for socioeconomic status, 13% of UP individuals attained higher education compared to 27.3% of the AP group. Conclusions at age 21 indicated that the UP children had been raised in unstable and less emotionally secure homes than the control subjects: "The most consistent difference noted, regardless of social grouping, was that UP children achieved a lower level of education than did the AP controls" (David et al. 1988, p. 43).

By the age of 35, institutional analysis indicated higher percentages of UP individuals in psychiatric consultation and hospitalization (43.3% UP, 30.8% AP), registration for crime or delinquency (23.3% UP, 16.7% AP), registration for drunken misconduct (20.8% UP, 12.5% AP), public assistance at ages 16–35 (25% UP, 15.8% AP), and subnormal educability or ineducability (10.8% UP, 5% AP). In the opposite direction was the finding that those not appearing on any registration list were 35% of UP individuals and 54.2% of AP control subjects. At age 35 there was a decrease in the difference between the two groups, but there were consistently more UP individuals than AP individuals with social and psychiatric problems.

In 1963, Czechoslovakia liberalized its abortion law, although there was still official sanction required, and individuals were denied permission to have an abortion for various reasons. An interested worker in the Bureau of Statistics kept the names of those who had been denied. Asking what would be the psychological results of unwantedness, H.P. David, Z. Dytryk, Z. Matecek, and V. Schuller undertook the Prague Study of children born to women who had twice been denied abortion for the same pregnancy. This longitudinal study of the 220 children was done with a control group matched for socioeconomic status, ethnic identity, and intelligence and drawn from the same schools. There were subtle differences in several levels of functioning at age 9: "They started life in conditions of physical and mental health similar to those of the AP children, but subsequently were breast-fed for shorter periods, were slightly but consistently overweight, and experienced a higher incidence of acute illness (and of longer duration for boys). While the intelligence of UP and AP children was normal, UP children had lower school grades. Their intellectual capabilities were less apparent in socially demanding situations" (David et al. 1988, p. 84). By age 22, as the subjects entered their own family-building years, clear differences were found between UP individuals (both females and males) and the control subjects, including increased rates of depression and psychiatric treatment. In addition, twice as many (23 UP, 11 AP) UP individuals already had criminal records. The individual costs of unwantedness noticeable in the early school years had accelerated during adolescence and early adulthood.

In another study, carried out in Santiago, Chile, where there is excellent and almost universal prenatal and well-baby care and abortion is illegal (Viel and Pereda 1988), 2,500 women were interviewed during prenatal care in the 6th or 7th month of pregnancy about whether the pregnancy was wanted, would be better at another time, or was unwanted. Home interviews were then undertaken when the infant was 3 months and 12 months of age. Twenty-nine percent of the women indicated that their pregnancy was unwanted. One finding of this study was that 81% of the wanted children were brought for their scheduled well-baby clinic appointments, whereas 68% of the unwanted group appeared. By 1 year of age there were noticeable differences in nutritional status between wanted and unwanted children, although food supplements were available to all. The authors concluded that "the percentage of undernourished children was higher for the unwanted babies in all socioeconomic groups compared to the wanted ones, indicating that the health of the child is related more to whether or not the pregnancy was wanted rather than to socioeconomic status" (Viel and Pereda 1988, p. 5), that differences in care are correlated in the first year of life with wantedness, and that unwantedness indicates problems of attachment and caring that are immediately visible.

The methods and timing of these studies differ, but they all show the importance of early social environment in human development and complex psychosocial problems associated with involuntary childbearing.

Conclusions

Within the biological context of reproduction, there is a kind of natural quality control—the early sloughing off of poorly paired chromosomes, the products of conception that are incompatible with life, or those that for various reasons are not implanted or that find an incompatible maternal chemical environment. This broad range of circumstances result in a basic reproductive failure rate of more than half. Historical differences in the definition of the beginning of life and reasons for this variation along with cross-cultural variation in social control of reproduction create environments in which differences in the meaning of kinship and continuity appear throughout the world. Indeed, such differences coexist in the modern world. Finally, unwanted children haunt city streets in the major urban centers of the world, and the costs to those who are born but not abandoned have become clear through carefully controlled research.

These descriptions are only samples of the rich variety of human response from the broad-based literatures of many disciplines. But these factors indicate widely varying responses to membership in and recruitment to society. Conclusions emerging from these descriptions are that less than half of all conceptions survive to viable birth; that unwanted children are at high risk for learning disability and compromised health; and that societies everywhere and always have defined life and controlled reproduction according to their own philosophical, religious, economic, and (most often) political principles.

References

Akhter HH, Rider R: Menstrual regulation v contraception in Bangladesh: characteristics of the acceptors. Studies in Family Planning 14:318, 1983

Basker E: The "natural" control of fertility. Sociology of Health and Illness 8(2):3–25, 1986

Boswell J: The Kindness of Strangers. New York, Pantheon, 1988

Brunt PA: Italian Manpower 225 BC to AD 14. London, Oxford University Press, 1971

Cook RJ, Dickens BM: International developments in abortion laws: 1977–88. Am J Public Health 78:1305–1311, 1988

David HP, Dytrych Z, Matejcek Z, et al (eds): Born Unwanted: Developmental Effects of Denied Abortion. New York, Springer, 1988

Dickison SK: Abortion in antiquity. Arethusa 6:159–166, 1973

Elias S, Annas GJ: Reproductive Genetics and the Law. Chicago, IL, Year Book Medical, 1987

Feen RH: Abortion and exposure in ancient Greece: assessing the status of the fetus and "newborn" from classical sources, in Abortion and the Status of the Fetus. Edited by Bondeson WB, Engelhardt HT Jr, Spicker SF, et al. Dordrecht, Holland, D Reidel, 1983

Forssman H, Thuwe I: Continued follow-up study of 120 persons born after refusal of application for therapeutic abortion. Acta Psychiatr Scand 64:142–146, 1981

Fuchs RG: Abandoned Children: Foundlings and Child Welfare in Nineteenth-Century France. Albany, NY, State University of New York Press, 1984

Gies F, Gies J: Marriage and the Family in the Middle Ages. New York, Harper & Row, 1987

Golden M: Demography and the exposure of girls at Athens. Phoenix 35:316–331, 1981

Henshaw SK, Silverman J: The characteristics and prior contraceptive use of U.S. abortion patients. Fam Plann Perspect 20:158–168, 1988

Karve I: Kinship Organization in India, Revised Edition. New York, Asia Publishing, 1965

Lederberg J: Experimental genetics and human evolution. American Naturalist 100:519–531, 1966

Luker K: Abortion and the Politics of Motherhood. Berkeley, University of California Press, 1984

McKeon R (ed): The Basic Works of Aristotle. Translated by Smith JA. New York, Random House, 1941

Newman LF: Abortion as folk medicine. California Health, October–November 1965, pp 75–79

Newman LF: Between the Ideal and Reality: Values in American Society: The Case for Legalized Abortion Now. Berkeley, CA, Diablo, 1967

Newman LF: Birth Control: An Anthropological View. Reading, MA, Addison-Wesley, 1972

Newman LF: Ophelia's herbal. Economic Botany 33:2, 1980

Newman LF (ed): Women's Medicine: A Cross-cultural Study of Indigenous Fertility Regulation. New Brunswick, NJ, Rutgers University Press, 1985

Ngin C: Indigenous fertility regulating methods among two Chinese communities in Malaysia, in Women's Medicine. Edited by Newman LF. New Brunswick, NJ, Rutgers University Press, 1985

Osofsky HJ: The Abortion Experience: Psychological and Mental Impact. New York, Harper & Row, 1973

Roberts CJ, Lowe CR: Where have all the conceptions gone? Lancet 1:498–499, 1975

Roe v. Wade, 410 U.S. 113 (1973)

Rosenberg M, Rochat R, Jabeen S, et al: Attitudes of rural Bangladesh physicians toward abortion. Studies in Family Planning 12:318–321, 1981

Shepard TH, Fantel AG: Embryonic and early fetal loss. Clin Perinatol 6:219–243, 1979

Symonds PV: Women and birth in the Hmong community. Paper presented at the annual meeting of the American Anthropological Association, Phoenix, AZ, November 1988

Veyne P (ed): A History of Private Life, Vol 1: From Pagan Rome to Byzantium. Translated by Goldhammer A. Cambridge, MA, Belknap Press, 1987

Viel B, Pereda C: Factors Associated With Birth of Unwanted Children and Risk in Health, Nutrition and Development That These Children Have During Their First Year of Life. Department of Health, University of Chile, 1988

Wasser SK: Infertility, abortion, and biotechnology. Human Nature 1(1):3–24, 1990

Chapter 4

The Law of Abortion and Contraception— Past and Present

Lynn T. Shepler, M.D.

On July 3, 1989, the U.S. Supreme Court voted to uphold sharp restrictions on abortion rights in an opinion that stopped just short of overturning its landmark 1973 decision legalizing abortion, *Roe v. Wade*. In *Webster v. Reproductive Health Services*, a plurality of the court voted to uphold a 1986 Missouri statute that declares "life begins at conception," restricts access of pregnant women to public facilities for abortion, and creates a statutory presumption of fetal viability at 20 weeks gestation. The statute's declaration that life begins at conception and the court's assertion that the "state's compelling interest in fetal life is equally compelling before viability" portends restrictions on first-trimester abortion and certain forms of contraceptives.

Supreme Court involvement in questions directly related to reproduction is a recent phenomenon. Beginning in 1961, in *Poe v. Ullman*, the Supreme Court has ruled on approximately 25 cases involving women's legal access to abortion and contraception.[1] The history of the law of contraception and abortion is intertwined, not simply during the nineteenth century, during which the law explicitly impaired women's access to contraception and abortion, but as still-evolving legal and scientific history. This is most apparent in the recent introduction of "contragestives" (e.g., RU-486, an abortifacient and hormone medication) and the implications for contraceptive restrictions in the Supreme Court's most recent decision, *Webster v. Reproductive Health Services*, in which the court failed to strike down the preamble of a Missouri statute that declares "human life should be protected from the moment of conception."

The Law of Abortion and Contraception: 1650–1820

Few people are aware that early abortion was considered a common-law right of women at the time of the U.S. Founding Fathers. At the time of the American Revolution, abortion was governed by the tradition of the British common law, which considered abortion until the time of quickening a common-law right of women.[2] For the first half of the nineteenth century, the judicial precedent governing abortion was an 1812 Massachusetts case, *Commonwealth v. Bangs*, in which the Massachusetts Supreme Court affirmed a woman's legal capacity to terminate her pregnancy prior to quickening.[3] After quickening, abortion was considered a crime, although it was punished less harshly than the destruction of a physically independent person.

Nineteenth-century American women commonly practiced abortion in their homes from information passed by word of mouth or obtained from home medical journals. Midwives possessed knowledge on how to "bring on the menses," and physicians possessed significant technical knowledge about terminating pregnancy through surgical and pharmaceutical means. In contrast to modern assumptions about the risks of abortion during the nineteenth century, by the medical standards of the day, abortion was considered relatively safe and certainly did not exceed the morbidity and mortality of childbirth.

Before 1820, no state barred women legal access to contraception or abortion before quickening. During the next 80 years, vocal members of the country's "regular" physicians, men who were white native-born Protestants and possessed formal medical training in the European tradition, fought to control the licensing of physicians in their drive for professionalization. These men, the white Anglo-Saxon Protestant physicians, formed a core of activists who, in 1847, founded the American Medical Association (AMA) and led the struggle to abolish the practices of abortion and contraception—practices of laywomen and their competitors, the midwives and medical "irregulars."

The Great Medical Crusade Against Abortion and Contraception

Physicians' efforts were central in the enactment of nineteenth-century antiabortion and anticontraceptive legislation. Historian James Mohr, in his study on U.S. abortion policy, concluded that "vigorous efforts of America's regular physicians [proved] in the long run to be the single most important factor in altering the legal policies towards abortion in this country. . . . Virtually every petition on the subject of abortion placed before a state legislature in the nineteenth century, for example, came either from a medical organization or from an individual physician."[4]

At the turn of the century, medicine was a poorly paid profession and few practicing physicians actually possessed formal medical training. Men who had received medical training in the highest tradition of the times, the "regulars," resented competing with other practitioners who, in their view, had no right to represent themselves as medical practitioners. These irregulars were considered to demean the profession and to depress financial remuneration for medical services because of their large numbers. Abortion, in the view of the medical regulars, represented the loss of a lucrative and steady stream of patients to their competitors, a recognition that provided one of the sparks for the nineteenth-century antiabortion movement.

Connecticut was the first state to enact legislation limiting abortion. In 1821, the Connecticut legislature passed a statute that closely resembled a poison-control act designed to protect women from unscrupulous peddlers of abortifacients. The New York legislature also focused on unscrupulous practitioners in its efforts to regulate surgical procedures and enacted an 1828 statute prohibiting abortion after quickening. The statute made the person who performed the abortion criminally liable but did not impose criminal liability on the woman who sought or underwent the abortion.

By 1840, approximately 10 states had enacted abortion restrictions. Nevertheless, in more than half of the states, women's common-law right to terminate a pregnancy before quickening prevailed. Women's access to abortion and contraception was cited as the cause for the marked decline in the birthrate among educated Protestant women, particularly married women, during the mid-nineteenth century. This prompted state legislators (who were predominantly white, male, and Protestant) to tighten restrictions on abortion—for example, the New York legislature in 1845 made a woman criminally liable for performing an abortion on herself or for seeking or submitting to an abortion. Under the 1845 revised statute, a woman could be imprisoned for as long as 3–4 months or fined not more than $1,000.

Restrictions on access to contraceptives soon followed. In 1847, concern about declining birthrates prompted the Massachusetts legislature to prohibit the distribution of contraceptives and the publishing, advertising, and circulation of birth-control information. The statute carried a penalty of imprisonment for not more than 3 years or a fine of $1,000. Many popular medical treatises of the time advanced the notion that contraception was the denial of the rightful function of sexual intercourse, human reproduction.[5]

Despite the movement during the mid-nineteenth century to limit women's access to abortion in some states, there was generally a great upsurge in the numbers of women seeking and obtaining abortions. Physicians decried the "non-infanto mania" that afflicted the nation's women.[6] The practice of abortion, considered a lucrative procedure for practitioners, became more open and obvious, and the competition for women patients increased among medical practitioners. Abortion was the sole livelihood for some practitioners and became one of the first medical specialties in American medical history.

During this period, women began to receive detailed instruction in human anatomy and physiology, which some physicians regarded as a major factor in the increase in abortions that began during the 1840s. Some regulars called for the termination of anatomical instruction, because women were becoming skilled enough to perform their own abortions. In addition, home abortion was supported by competition among pharmaceutical houses, such as Parke-Davis, in the sale and marketing of autoabortive instruments and abortifacients.

During this period, the first American feminist movement was rising in stature and members of the medical regulars counted among the most virulent antifeminists of the late nineteenth century. In 1869 a medical crusader against abortion wrote: "Woman's rights and woman's sphere are, as understood by the American public, quite different from that understood by us as Physicians, or as Anatomists, or Physiologists." Mohr found that medical regulars, informed by their knowledge of physiology and embryology, viewed women's role in society to be solely a function of procreation: "To many doctors the chief purpose of women was to produce children; anything that interfered with that purpose, or allowed women to 'indulge' themselves in less important activities, threatened marriage, the family, and the future of society itself. Abortion was a supreme example of such an interference for these physicians."

Dr. Horatio Robinson Storer, the son of a Harvard obstetrician and gynecologist and himself a practitioner in obstetrics and gynecology, was one of the most prominent leaders in the regulars' drive for professionalization and crusade against abortion. Storer was "an outspoken opponent of new social roles for women," stating that "in loosing, as I hope to do, some of women's chains, it is solely for professional purposes, to increase her health, prolong her life, extend the benefits she confers upon society—in a word, selfishly to enhance her value to ourselves."[7] Storer also fought the entry of women into medicine and opposed liberal divorce laws.

During this period, many regulars composed treatises stating that the influx of Roman Catholic immigrants and their unrestrained breeding would result in reverse Darwinism, ruining the nation. Storer, too, expressed concern about Catholic immigration and stressed in his treatises that members of the Roman Catholic church did not practice abortion.

In contrast to the twentieth-century antiabortion movement, organized religion was not active in the political battle to criminalize abortion; nor was the nineteenth-century antiabortion movement a result of a ground-swell of public protest. Most citizens and religious clergy were uncon-cerned. At a gathering of Michigan regulars, one speaker declared, "It is not sufficient that the medical profession should set up a standard of morality for themselves, but the people are to be educated up to it."[8]

Regulars were generally contemptuous of the religious clergy for their failure to recognize the sin of abortion and physician's moral authority on the issue of abortion. The regulars received little organized support from the Roman Catholic Church. In 1869, however, Bishop Spaulding released a statement condemning abortion: "No mother is allowed under any cir-cumstances, to permit the death of her unborn infant, not even for the sake of preserving her own life." Regular physicians were dissatisfied with Spaulding's position because it did not contain the "therapeutic exception," an exception important to physicians as an expression of deference to physicians' moral and professional judgment.[9]

Most abortion legislation in existence in states immediately before *Roe v. Wade* was enacted during the 20-year span from 1860 to 1880. This political success of the regulars has been attributed to several factors. After Joseph Lister's breakthrough in the field of antisepsis in 1865, medicine became more respectable, expanding the regulars' influence in the political process. In addition, the Republican party, which rose to power during the postwar period, desired a more systematic approach to public policy and was more open to the influence of medical professionals. After 1870, "the regulars began to dominate and outdistance most of their rivals."[10]

During the postwar period, medical societies intensified their petitioning of state legislatures, resulting in increasingly restrictive statutes limiting abortion and contraception. In several state legislatures, much of the at-tention was focused on the actions of married women and the fall in the birth rate. Mohr noted, "Since one of the chief purposes of marriage was to ensure the procreation and proper upbringing of children, a woman who entered marriage could have no legitimate excuse for trying to ter-minate a pregnancy unless her life itself was actually at stake. The un-married aborter, on the other hand, as the innocent victim of seduction, would, in her understandable desperation, be permitted to retain her long-standing exemption from punishment."[11]

The regulars also limited their interaction with female physicians and refused to allow female practitioners to join their principal professional organization, the AMA. In 1868, the AMA rejected a proposal that would have permitted female practitioners to interact with regulars. In 1871, a proposal that would have permitted membership of female practitioners was likewise rejected.

Before the federal Comstock Act of 1873, all legislation restricting abortion and contraception was enacted in state legislatures. The Comstock Act, enacted by the U.S. Congress as part of the antiobscenity campaign by Anthony Comstock, prohibited the sale and importation of articles for the prevention of conception within all areas of federal jurisdiction, including the District of Columbia. Physicians were not exempt. It was not until 1936 that the Second Circuit Court of Appeals interpreted the act to exclude physicians in a legal challenge brought by a female gynecologist seeking to import vaginal pessaries.[12]

Legislation limiting women's access to abortion and contraception was eventually enacted in every state of the union with little opposition. Legislative and judicial challenges during the late 1800s and early 1900s were unsuccessful and appear to have focused on contraceptive restrictions.[13]

In examining judicial opinions issued during the last two centuries, it is remarkable that the abstract principle that women have a right to life and health has never been explicitly recognized as a basis for constitutional protection.[14] In *Tileston v. Ullman* (1943), the Connecticut Supreme Court went so far as to declare that the Connecticut legislature's failure to amend the anticontraception statute indicated that there were no implied exceptions to the statute even when pregnancy jeopardized a woman's life.[15] The case was appealed to the U.S. Supreme Court, which dismissed the case, noting that the plaintiff's sole constitutional attack was based on the deprivation of life of his patients, which the Court determined to be an insufficient basis on which to challenge the statute.

In *Roe v. Wade*, a married woman suffering from an underlying medical ailment and alleging that pregnancy would jeopardize her health was denied standing because the Supreme Court found her injury to be "too speculative." What the Court appeared to recognize and then dismiss is the risk of injury associated with heterosexual intercourse, which is imposed, to a greater or lesser degree, on almost all female partners in a heterosexual couple. Outside of rape and incest, no court has recognized that heterosexual intercourse is associated with physical risk for women.[16]

In his study of U.S. abortion policy, Mohr concluded that nineteenth-century abortion legislation was the real aberration of U.S. public policy on abortion. The highly charged issue of fetal life, alive in antiabortion sentiment today, was not what drove the antiabortion movement of the nineteenth century. Stated Mohr, "Regular physicians in the nineteenth century exploited the issue of abortion for a number of reasons of their own . . . yet the policy they established—a nearly absolute defense of fetal life at every stage of gestation—appears to have interested them only secondarily."[17]

Sexual Freedom and the Right to Privacy

Statutes restricting contraceptive use and distribution remained the law until the late 1960s. In the 1968 case of *Griswold v. Connecticut*, the U.S.

Supreme Court declared laws restricting the use of contraceptives by married couples to be an unconstitutional state infringement of personal privacy and liberty. The protection of access to contraception to the unmarried was extended in *Eisenstadt v. Baird* (1972), in which a Massachusetts statute prohibiting the distribution of contraceptives to unmarried persons was declared unconstitutional by the Supreme Court under the Equal Protection Clause.

As late as 1977, the state of New York sought to continue enforcement of its anticontraception statute, which restricted the advertising and sale of nonprescription contraceptives. The statute was declared unconstitutional in *Carey v. Population Services International* (1977), notable for the dissenting remarks of Justice William Rehnquist: If the men who "valiantly but vainly defended the heights of Bunker Hill . . . [knew] that their efforts had enshrined in the Constitution the right of commercial vendors of contraceptives to unmarried minors through such means as window displays and vending machines located in the men's room of truck stops . . . it is not difficult to imagine their reaction." Rehnquist contrasted the realm of the sacred (constitutional principles) with that of the profane (contraceptives). Not surprisingly, Rehnquist could find no principle under which to declare such restrictions on nonprescription contraceptives a violation of constitutional principles.[18]

While laws related to contraception were either repealed or enjoined during the late 1960s, a few states began to liberalize their abortion statutes, notably California and New York. Successful challenges to antiabortion statutes were also occurring in a handful of states, and some people have criticized the Supreme Court for failing to wait for the development of lower-court case law, which might have provided a more doctrinally mature analysis of the constitutional grounds for abortion rights.[19]

The Legalization of Abortion: *Roe v. Wade*

On January 22, 1972, in *Roe v. Wade*, the U.S. Supreme Court struck down a nineteenth-century Texas statute prohibiting abortion at all stages of pregnancy unless the life of the mother was threatened. Justice Harry Blackmun, writing for the majority, based the Court's holding on the existence of a "right to privacy" grounded in the notion of personal liberty protected by the Due Process Clause of the Fourteenth Amendment. The court situated the "fundamental decision whether to bear or beget a child" in a long line of decisions dating from the 1920s related to guarantees of personal privacy in matters related to marriage, childrearing, contraception, and family relationships.[20]

The question of fetal personhood was not decided by the Supreme Court; however, the Court stated that "if personhood is established" the woman's case "collapses, for the fetus' right to life would then be guaranteed specifically by the [Fourteenth] Amendment."[21] Antiabortion activists have attempted through the federal Human Life Amendment and declarations such as that found in the Missouri preamble in *Webster* to build a legal foundation for a reversal of *Roe v. Wade* on the theory of fetal personhood.[22]

As a matter of constitutional law, restrictions on the exercise of fundamental right may be based only on a compelling state interest. When a fundamental right is implicated, the court uses "strict scrutiny" in determining whether an infringement of a fundamental right is "narrowly tailored" and "reasonably related" to the state's compelling interest. When a fundamental right is not implicated, a lower standard of judicial review or "scrutiny" is used—"rational basis" review, which is generally used in cases of economic or social regulation. Under the rational basis test, the issue then becomes whether a legislative restriction bears "some rational relationship to legitimate state interests."*

In the cases that followed *Roe*, the Supreme Court at times appeared to use "strict scrutiny," although using the language of "unduly burdensome" (i.e., a statute is unconstitutional if it unduly burdens a woman's ability to exercise her constitutional right). Note that the standard of review that the court elects to use ("strict scrutiny" versus "rational basis" review) is often critical to the outcome of a case—which will become more obvious in my discussion of the *Webster* decision.

In *Roe*, the Supreme Court recognized two compelling state interests that justified state regulation of abortion—maternal health and fetal life, which the Court held were demarcated by the trimesters of pregnancy. Viability was held to mark the beginning of the "state's compelling interest in fetal life," and the end of the first trimester—the point at which mortality from abortion approaches that of childbirth—was determined to be the point at which the state has a compelling interest in protecting maternal health.[23]

Subsequent to *Roe*, regulations creating an "absolute obstacle" to abortion have been declared unconstitutional. A statute permitting a male spouse or a parent to have absolute veto power over a woman's decision to undergo an abortion creates an absolute obstacle and is thus unconstitutional.[24] In the case of minors, the Supreme Court has required states to provide an alternative procedure, also called a "judicial bypass," through which a minor may demonstrate that she is mature enough to make the abortion decision or that "despite her immaturity, an abortion would be in her best interests."[25]

First-trimester abortion has been judged to be solely the province of a

---

*These specific phrases (i.e., "strict scrutiny," "rational basis," etc.) are used in Supreme Court opinions to indicate the technical process of constitutional decision making. The level of "scrutiny" that the Court elects to utilize often appears to determine the outcome of a case.

woman and her physician. Regulation is permitted only to the extent that regulations have "no significant impact on the woman's exercise of her right" or, where justified, by "important state health objectives."[26] Limits on first-trimester abortion held permissible by the Supreme Court include the requirement that a woman give written informed consent to the procedure, that the abortion be performed by a licensed physician, and that tissue specimens obtained during the abortion be submitted for a pathology report. Physicians may also be required to keep certain records of the procedure and the patient.[27]

Before the *Webster* decision, regulation of second-trimester abortions was based on the "state's compelling interest in maternal health," which was declared to begin at the end of the first trimester, the point at which mortality rates of first-trimester abortion approached those of childbirth. Based on this rationale, states have been permitted to regulate abortion in ways reasonably related to maternal health consistent with accepted medical practice. State restrictions on second-trimester abortions have been declared unconstitutional by the Supreme Court when regulations increased cost or limited the availability of abortion without promoting important health benefits, such as the requirement that all second-trimester abortions be performed in hospitals.[28]

Based on a "state's compelling interest in potential life," after viability the state may, "if it chooses, regulate, and even proscribe, abortion except where it is necessary, in appropriate medical judgment, for the preservation of the life, or health of the mother."[29] The Supreme Court has upheld restrictions on abortions after viability, which have included the requirement that two physicians be present during postviability abortions and, most recently in the *Webster* case, the statutory presumption of viability at 20 weeks, which a physician must rebut before performing an abortion.[30]

Although the Supreme Court has upheld the requirement that a woman provide informed consent to the abortion, the Court has declared statutory "informed consent" requirements unconstitutional when a state mandates the physician to read a "parade of horribles" to the pregnant woman—regardless of the circumstances surrounding the abortion. In the words of Justice Lewis Powell, "The States are not free, under the guise of protecting maternal health of potential life, to intimidate women into continuing pregnancies."[31] The informed consent function may not be used "to influence the woman's informed choice between abortion or childbirth"; nor can it be used to place "obstacles in the path of the doctor" performing the abortion. Until the *Webster* case, the Court has protected the physician-patient relationship and permitted physicians to control the information that, in the physician's judgment, is needed by the patient to make an informed decision. This is likely to change under the Rehnquist Court.[32] Among other provisions that the Court has invalidated are a state ban on abortion advertising,[33] a city regulation mandating a 24-hour waiting period before an abortion,[34] and a state regulation establishing hospital committees for approving women's abortion requests.[35]

The Abortion-Funding Cases: Rational-Basis Review

The U.S. Supreme Court has uniformly upheld stringent state and federal abortion-funding restrictions. In these cases, the Court has used its least-stringent mode of judicial review (i.e., the "rationality" review) and has expressed the view that states may make policy judgments favoring "normal" childbirth over abortion—even when a woman's health may be permanently jeopardized as a result of carrying a pregnancy to term. Not surprisingly, these opinions have provoked sharp dissent from the Court's more liberal members.[36]

In *Harris v. McRae*, the most restrictive of the funding decisions, the Supreme Court upheld the Hyde Amendment, which permits states to refuse Medicaid coverage for "medically necessary" abortions, even when the continuance of the pregnancy may result in severe permanent damage to a woman's health. The Hyde Amendment limits abortion coverage to cases in which the woman's life is endangered by the pregnancy or the woman was impregnated by an act of rape or incest.[37]

Restrictions on abortion funding have been upheld under the principle that although indigence may be an "absolute obstacle" to abortion, it is not an obstacle of a state's creation. With this rationale, the Supreme Court has held that funding childbirth but not abortion does not unduly burden a woman's exercise of her constitutional right, even when indigence makes obtaining an abortion a virtual impossibility. One of the most disturbing questions in these cases is whether the state may condition the grant of medical benefits on the recipient's relinquishment of her constitutional rights. Precedents involving questions other than abortion suggest that this is unconstitutional.[38] Another major issue is whether this denial of benefits constitutes an equal protection violation because, in the words of Justice Thurgood Marshall, "the cruel impact falls exclusively on indigent pregnant women" who are also disproportionately African American, Hispanic, or members of other racial groups.[39]

Before the *Webster* decision, the Supreme Court specifically reaffirmed *Roe v. Wade* in its decision in *Akron* (1983) and *Thornburgh* (1986). Justice Powell, writing for the majority in *Akron*, warned of the views eventually articulated by the Rehnquist Court in *Webster*. Powell stated that the dissent of Justices Sandra O'Connor, Byron White, and Rehnquist "does not think that even one of the numerous abortion regulations at issue imposes a sufficient burden on the 'limited' fundamental right to require heightened scrutiny." Powell noted that the dissent adopted the rational-basis test, inconsistent "with the existence of a fundamental right recognized in *Roe v. Wade.*" The dissent, he warned, adopted reasoning that, "for all practice purposes," would overrule *Roe.*[40]

Six years later, in *Webster v. Reproductive Health Services* (1989), a newly constituted conservative majority began dismantling the Supreme Court's decade and a half history of protecting abortion rights.

Abortion and the Rehnquist Court:
Webster v. Reproductive Health Services

Missouri has, since the case of *Roe v. Wade*, sought to limit women's access to abortion through legislative restrictions that were later declared unconstitutional by the U.S. Supreme Court in *Planned Parenthood of Missouri v. Danforth* (1976) and *Planned Parenthood Assn. of Kansas City v. Ashcroft* (1983). In 1989, after a lower federal court declared Missouri's most recent abortion statute unconstitutional, the Supreme Court's newly constituted conservative majority reached out to rehabilitate the 1986 Missouri abortion statute in the case *Webster v. Reproductive Health Services*, in a decision that suggests a radical reversal in Supreme Court jurisprudence on abortion.

In a 5-to-4 ruling authored by Chief Justice Rehnquist, the Supreme Court upheld four provisions of the Missouri statute: 1) a statutory presumption of fetal viability at 20 weeks, which a physician may rebut through the performance of certain tests that are, in the physician's judgment, indicated to determine the viability of the fetus; 2) the legislative finding that "life begins at conception"; 3) prohibition of the use of public employees and facilities to perform or assist with abortions not necessary to save the mother's life; 4) prohibition of the use of public funds, employees, or facilities for encouraging or counseling a woman to have an abortion not necessary to save her life. In addition, the Court gutted *Roe*'s trimester framework, which portends future decisions in which the Court may rescind constitutional protection for women's access to first-trimester abortion and certain forms of contraception.

Standard of Review: The Rational-Basis Test

In sharp contrast to previous U.S. Supreme Court analysis of abortion restrictions, the Court deciding the *Webster* case applied the least-rigorous standard of review, which permitted the Court to uphold the Missouri statute, which likely would have fallen—either in its entirety or in its separate provisions—under a more rigorous standard of scrutiny. The plurality abandoned fundamental-rights analysis and proposed a new standard with which to judge the constitutionality of state abortion restrictions—whether the legislation "permissibly furthers the State's interest in protecting potential human life."[41]

Through the use of the lowest tier of judicial scrutiny, the Supreme Court implicitly repudiates its finding in *Roe v. Wade* that the decision whether to bear a child is a fundamental right. As Justice Blackmun pointed out in his dissent, "The plurality's novel test appears to be nothing more than a dressed-up version of rational-basis review, this Court's most lenient level of scrutiny. One thing is clear, however: were the plurality's permissibly furthers standard adopted by the Court, for all practical purposes, *Roe* would be overruled."

The Supreme Court provides no guidance as to what it considers the constitutional limits of this lower standard of review—in essence, inviting an avalanche of antiabortion legislation designed to test the constitutional parameters of the Court's revised standard.

Trimester Analysis: "A Virtual Procrustean Bed"

The *Webster* plurality jettisoned the Supreme Court's traditional trimester analysis, declaring that the "rigid" trimester analysis made the constitutional law of abortion "a virtual Procrustean bed." Chief Justice Rehnquist (joined by Justices White and Anthony Kennedy) stated that he could find no reason why the state's interest in potential life "should come into existence only at the point of viability. . . . The State's interest, if compelling after viability, is equally compelling before viability."

Denouncing the plurality opinion, Justice Blackmun accused the plurality of creating a "contrived conflict" for instituting a "radical reversal of the law of abortion." In his view, the Missouri statute could have been upheld under the *Roe* trimester analysis, but the Supreme Court aggressively reinterprets the state's interest—now held to be "compelling" before viability—to justify its abandonment of the trimester framework. While agreeing with Blackmun that there was no need to scuttle *Roe*'s trimester analysis, Justice O'Connor shared the plurality's reading of the language of the statute and voted with Rehnquist to uphold the statutory presumption of viability at 20 weeks of gestation.

Whether the plurality would recognize restrictions on first-trimester abortion or permit state protection of the newly fertilized ovum is unclear. Abandonment of *Roe*'s trimester analysis is significant because it formed part of the constitutional framework protecting women's access to first- and second-trimester abortion. Although abortion may remain a fundamental right in theory, if the state's compelling interest in potential life may permissibly begin at fertilization or during the first trimester, this will permit recriminalization of abortion at all stages of pregnancy and provide a basis for restricting forms of contraception that act after fertilization.

The Missouri Preamble: "Life Begins at Conception"

An *unborn child* is defined in the 1986 Missouri statute as "the offspring of human beings from the moment of conception until birth and at every stage of its biological development, including the human conceptus, zygote, morula, blastocyst, embryo, and fetus." According to the statute, conception is "the fertilization of the ovum of a female by a sperm of a male."

Declarations of when life begins have been found unconstitutional in previous Supreme Court decisions when used to justify abortion restrictions. Asserting that a "state may not adopt one theory of when life begins to justify its regulation of abortions," the Supreme Court, in *Akron v. Akron Center for Reproductive Health* (1983), declared unconstitutional an Akron ordinance stating that life begins at the "union of sperm and egg."[42] In marked contrast, Chief Justice Rehnquist finds that the Missouri preamble expresses a permissible "value judgment favoring childbirth over abortion" allowable under *Roe*. Citing the *Akron* "dicta," Rehnquist interprets *Akron* to mean that state declarations about the beginning of life may not be used to justify a constitutionally invalid abortion restriction but that there is no constitutional impediment for a state to use a definition of life to justify a constitutionally valid abortion restriction. Rehnquist finds that the preamble merely provides "protections to unborn children in tort and probate law," and it "can be interpreted to do no more than that." Because the preamble imposes "no substantive restrictions on abortion," the plurality concludes that it need not pass on the question of its constitutionality.

In dissent, Justice Blackmun (joined by Justices William Brennan and Marshall) found that the preamble "unconstitutionally burdens the use of contraceptive devices such as the IUD [intrauterine device] and the 'morning after' pill, which may operate to prevent pregnancy only after conception." Justice John Paul Stevens went farther, arguing that the preamble violates the Establishment Clause of the First Amendment because it expresses a theological definition of human life. Stevens perceptively noted that the Missouri statute reflects the historical conflict between the definition of *conception* by the American College of Obstetricians and Gynecologists and the definition of *conception* by the National Right to Life Committee and others, including the Roman Catholic Church.[43] Stevens stated:

> The Missouri statute defines "conception" as "the fertilization of the ovum of a female by a sperm of a male" even though standard medical tests equate "conception" with implantation in the uterus, occurring about six days after fertilization. Missouri's declaration therefore implies regulation not only of previability abortions, but also of common forms of contraception such as the IUD and the morning after pill.

It is important to recognize that the definition of life contained in the Missouri statute is a particular political and theological definition of life, which such groups as the National Right to Life Committee, Catholics United for Life, and the American Life League have tailored for the advancement of their goal to limit access to particular forms of contraception and abortion.[44]

Restrictions on Public Employees and Facilities Upheld

Under the principle enunciated in the abortion-funding cases that the Due Process Clause "generally confers no affirmative right to governmental aid, even where such aid may be necessary to secure life, liberty, or property interests," the Court deciding the *Webster* case upheld the restrictions placed on public employees and the use of public facilities for performing abortions.

The Supreme Court reasoned that "the State's decision . . . to use public facilities and staff to encourage childbirth over abortion places no governmental obstacle in the path of a woman who chooses to terminate her pregnancy." The Missouri statute also contains a provision that prohibited public employees (including physicians) from counseling women. Missouri did not appeal this ruling in its case before the Supreme Court. It is an issue that may affect all physicians by opening the door for state-mandated "gag orders" that require physicians to practice state medicine under the force of criminal or civil penalties, including loss of licensure.

Abortion: A Political Question

Obviously, restrictions on physician-patient dialogue have profound implications for the practice of psychiatry. Under some circumstances, a psychiatrist may be under a legal and ethical obligation to discuss abortion as an option—for example, when a patient has been treated with psychotropic medications before pregnancy was diagnosed or when she has suffered severe psychiatric decompensations following previous deliveries.

Although the plurality opinion contains remarks suggesting that the Supreme Court views questions of abortion regulation to be a matter of political debate and not constitutional adjudication, none are so virulent as the remarks of Justice Antonin Scalia, who attacked his fellow justices, particularly Justice O'Connor, for their failure to use *Webster* as a vehicle for overturning *Roe*. Arguing that questions concerning women's control over their reproductive functions are a function of the "popular will," Scalia stated that "the answers to most of the cruel questions posed are political and not juridical. . . ."[45]

In retort, Justice Blackmun argued that abortion rights belong to the realm not subject to the vagaries of political processes: "The very purpose of a Bill of Rights was to withdraw certain subjects from the vicissitudes of political controversy, to place them beyond the reach of majorities and officials and to establish them as legal principles to be applied by the Courts. One's right[s] to life, liberty, and property . . . may not be submitted to vote; they depend on the outcome of no election."[46]

The Supreme Court's factions clearly hold sharply contrasting visions of the nature of abortion rights. It is remarkable, given the tremendous legal and social importance of the *Webster* decision, that so little reasoning was provided by the plurality to support its decision. In the words of Blackmun, "The opinion contains not one word of rationale for its view of the State's interest. This it-is-so-because-we-say-so jurisprudence constitutes nothing other than an attempted exercise of brute force: reason, much less persuasion, has no place."

The Effects of the *Webster* Decision

The success of the *Webster* case is anticipated to spur the Missouri legislature to draft new legislation containing tighter restrictions on abortion. Under the leadership of Missouri Governor John Ashcroft, it is expected that there will be new legislative action to prohibit abortion in all cases, including rape and incest.[47]

After the *Webster* decision, two medical centers were ordered to cease performing abortions, Truman Medical Center in Kansas City and University Hospital in Columbia, Missouri—the only facilities outside St. Louis where women may obtain abortions after the 12th week of pregnancy. This ban is anticipated to affect poor women most severely.[48] One example of the effects of the restriction is revealed in a report of a woman who was forced to travel 250 miles to another state to terminate her pregnancy with an anencephalic fetus.

Interpretation of the statute's preamble has had unexpected effects. Although Chief Justice Rehnquist declared the preamble of the Missouri statute to be simply a "value judgment" with no operative effect on limiting women's access to abortion, a St. Louis County Circuit Court judge used the preamble to acquit 11 antiabortion protesters charged with criminal trespass. On August 16, 1989, Judge George Gerhard cited the preamble in recognizing the demonstrators' defense of necessity in unlawfully entering the abortion clinic. In his acquittal of the demonstrators, the judge stated that the "violations were necessary as emergency measures to avoid the death and maiming of unborn children."

The U.S. Supreme Court: The Future of Abortion Rights

The Missouri statute upheld in *Webster* limited women's access to public hospitals, where only a minority of abortions are performed. More serious challenges to abortion rights are anticipated in the Supreme Court's 1990 term, in which the court has agreed to hear cases that present the opportunity to recognize restriction on first-trimester abortion.[49] Many believe that the Court will uphold restrictions on abortion based on the lower standard of review, which will effectively overrule *Roe*.

The voting record of the members of the Supreme Court's conservative majority lends support to the view that the Court will uphold severe restrictions on women's access to abortion. Chief Justice Rehnquist has voiced consistent antipathy for the notion of constitutionally based reproductive rights, including the right to freedom from state interference in the use or sale of contraceptives.[50] His views appear to be unchanged since his dissent in *Roe* in 1973 and are reflected virtually without alteration in his plurality opinion in *Webster*.[51]

Examples of severe restrictions on abortion that have been supported by members of the Supreme Court's conservative majority include legislation giving husbands absolute veto power over a wife's decision to undergo an abortion, regardless of the state of the marriage (Rehnquist, White); legislation giving a parent absolute veto power over a daughter's decision to undergo an abortion, regardless of whether she was a victim of incest or rape or the state of the parent-child relationship (Rehnquist, White); legislation making physicians guilty of manslaughter when a physician fails "to preserve the life and health of the fetus" while performing an abortion" [*sic*] (Rehnquist, White); legislation requiring all second-trimester abortions to be performed in hospitals (Rehnquist, White, O'Connor); legislation requiring physicians to read coercive and intimidating informed-consent provisions to patients (Rehnquist, White, O'Connor); and legislation requiring 24-hour waiting periods after a woman seeks an abortion (Rehnquist, White, O'Connor).[52]

The Supreme Court and Abortifacients

Few people are aware that legislation in the wake of *Roe* has also included attempts to regulate women's access to abortifacient contraceptives.[53] Abortifacient contraceptives were the focus of the Supreme Court case of *Diamond v. Charles*, 476 U.S. 54 (1986), in which the Court let stand a lower federal court decision enjoining an Illinois statute that subjected physicians to criminal penalties for their failure to inform a patient that the prescription the physician prescribed was an abortifacient. It is unclear how the Supreme Court would rule on the issue of abortifacients; however, it is clear that organized political opposition exists to limit their use and development.

"Microabortion" is the term used by Dr. Jack Wilke, president of the National Right to Life Committee and a devout Roman Catholic, in describing the antigestational effects of low-dose oral contraceptives and the IUD.[54] He also described the actions of diethylstilbestrol administered to a rape victim who had been impregnated: "The drug had hardened the lining of the womb. About one week after fertilization, the multicelled tiny boy or girl could not implant and died. This mechanism was an abortion."[55]

Other major figures in the antiabortion movement have also expressed their opposition to the use of contraception. Randall Terry, the organizer of Operation Rescue, wrote, "I don't think Christians should use birth control. You consummate your marriage as often as you like and if you have babies, you have babies." Abortifacients are attacked in literature distributed by state chapters of the National Right to Life Committee: "The Birth Control Pill Kills Babies"; "Is Your 'Contraceptive' Really Killing Babies?"; "Oral Contraceptives: The Medical Evidence for Covert Abortion"; "The Pill and the IUD as Abortifacients"; "The Case for Natural Family Planning."[56]

Public policies establishing protections for zygotes are obviously more ominous than earlier antiabortion legislation. In contrast to the nineteenth-century rationales for the criminalization of abortion, which had as their alleged focus the health and well-being of women, twentieth-century rationales that have as their focus the compulsory gestation of fetal life inevitably lead to the position that it is not simply an issue of whether states criminalize abortion and abortifacient contraceptives, but that they base their decisions on the protection accorded persons under the Fourteenth Amendment. Thus twentieth-century abortion legislation is potentially more restrictive and punitive than earlier legislation.

Among antiabortion advocates during the nineteenth and twentieth centuries, physicians have been the principal targets for prosecution.[57] Physicians must anticipate more restrictions on contraception and abortion, which will have a direct impact on medical practice and will carry criminal or civil penalties for physician noncompliance, including the threat of loss of licensure or imprisonment. The exact trajectory on abortion rights of the Supreme Court's new conservative majority is unclear, but in the words of Justice Blackmun in *Webster*, "the signs are evident and very ominous, and a chill wind blows."[58]

Notes

1. *Poe v. Ullman*, 367 U.S. 497 (1961); *Griswold v. Connecticut*, 381 U.S. 479 (1965); *Eisenstadt v. Baird*, 405 U.S. 438 (1972); *Roe v. Wade*, 410 U.S. 113 (1973); *Doe v. Bolton*, 410 U.S. 179 (1973); *Bigelow v. Virginia*, 421 U.S. 809 (1975); *Connecticut v. Menillo*, 423 U.S. 9 (1975); *Singleton v. Wulff*, 428 U.S. 106 (1976); *Planned Parenthood of Missouri v. Danforth*, 428 U.S. 52 (1976); *Bellotti v. Baird (I)*, 428 U.S. 132 (1976); *Carey v. Population Services International*, 431 U.S. 678 (1977); *Beal v. Doe*, 432 U.S. 438 (1977); *Maler v. Roe*, 432 U.S. 464 (1977); *Poelker v. Doe* 432 U.S. 519 (1977); *Colautti v. Franklin*, 439 U.S. 379 (1979); *Belotti v. Baird (II)*, 443 U.S. 622 (1979); *Harris v. McRae*, 448 U.S. 297 (1980); *Williams v. Zbaraz*, 448 U.S. 358 (1980); *H.L. v. Matheson*, 450 U.S. 398 (1981); *Akron v. Akron Center for Reproductive Health*, 462

U.S. 416 (1983); *Planned Parenthood Assn. of Kansas City v. Ashcroft*, 462 U.S. 476 (1983); *Simopoulos v. Virginia*, 462 U.S. 506 (1983); *Diamond v. Charles*, 106 S.Ct. 1697 (1986); *Thornburgh v. American College of Obstetricians and Gynecologists*, 106 S.Ct. 2169 (1986); *Webster v. Reproductive Health Services*, 109 S.Ct. 3040 (1989)

2. Mohr JC: Abortion in America: The Origins and Evolution of National Policy, 1800–1900. Oxford, UK, Oxford University Press, 1978, p vii. Quickening was the point, late in the fourth or fifth months, at which time a woman could sense fetal movement.

3. 9 Mass. 387 (1812)

4. Mohr (1978), p 261

5. Ball C: Female sexual ideologies in mid to late nineteenth-century Canada. Canadian Journal of Women and the Law 1:324–338, 1986

6. Mohr (1978), p 168

7. Storer, cited in Mohr (1978), p 169

8. E.P. Christian cited in Mohr (1978), p 171

9. The nineteenth-century struggle around abortion is similar to that of the twentieth century in the sense that the issue is not whether the decision itself can be made (to abort) but who makes the decision. In both centuries, the battle was pitted between women and antifeminist factions.

10. Mohr (1978), p 204

11. Mohr (1978), p 209

12. *United States v. One Package*, 86 F.2d 737 (2d Cir 1936)

13. Some attempts were made to challenge these statutes in the courts. See *State v. Nelson*, 126 Conn. 412, 11 A.2d 856 (1940) (the Connecticut Supreme Court declared an anticontraception statute constitutional) and *Tileston v. Ullman*, 129 Conn. 84, 26 A.2d 582 (1942) (the Connecticut Supreme Court reaffirmed the constitutionality of the Connecticut anticontraception statute).

For historical interest see *People v. Byrne*, 99 Misc. 1, 163 N.Y. Supp. 682 (Sup. Ct. Kings County 1917) (state prosecution of Margaret Sanger after she was charged with distributing a pamphlet entitled "What Every Girl Should Know") and *People v. Sanger*, 222 N.Y. 192, 118 N.E. 637 (1918) (state prosecution of Margaret Sanger for distributing contraception information). See also *Baretta v. Baretta*, 182 Misc. 852, 46 N.Y.S.2d 261 (Sup. Ct. Queens County 1944) (action by wife for marital separation for husband's refusal to use a contraceptive, in which the court dismissed the wife's complaint stating that it was a wife's obligation to have sexual relations with her husband and that the use of contraceptives was contrary to the public policy of the state of New York).

Other state courts entertained challenges to state anticontraception statutes beginning in the 1920s and ending with the declaration by the U.S. Supreme Court in 1968 that these statutes' unconstitutionality abridged an individual's "right to privacy." Until then, no state court recognized a woman's or couple's right to use contraception.

Other cases were tested challenging federal anticontraception laws, particularly the Comstock Act: *Youngs Rubber Corp v. C.I. Lee & Co.*, 45 F.2d 103 (2d Cir 1930); *Davis v. United States*, 62 F.2d 473 (6th Cir. 1933); *United States v. One Package*, 13 F. Supp. 334 (S.D.N.Y.), aff'd, 86 F.2d 737 (2d Cir. 1936) (woman gynecologist imported vaginal pessaries for research purposes to be employed to save the life or to promote the physical well-being of women patients, which the Second Circuit held not be barred by the Comstock Act).

14. In twentieth-century decisions, rights to abortion and contraception are cast in the paler constitutional versions of "privacy" or, at best, procreational choice. The U.S. Supreme Court has never elaborated on the constitutional underpinnings

of these rights and has gone so far as to repudiate that these rights are based on notions of bodily integrity (which some argue to be one of the principle constitutional grounds for abortion rights). Couching the nature of abortion rights as a matter of procreational choice only, the Court appears to view pregnancy as "natural" and ignores the medical risks associated with undertaking even a "normal" pregnancy. This is particularly remarkable given the degree to which the Court's opinions are medicalized. Feminists have criticized modern obstetrics for perpetuating the view that pregnancy is pathological or dangerous and involves numerous medical risks that can only be attended to by qualified physicians. It is remarkable that Supreme Court jurisprudence solidly incorporates the medical perspective of pregnancy with this notable exception. It is also remarkable that the court has chosen to seize this particular aspect of women's "normal" reproductive functions: the "normal period" could just as easily serve as a focus, with pregnancy viewed as its interruption. See *Poelker v. Doe*, 432 U.S. 519, 522 (1977) ("We merely hold . . . that the Constitution does not forbid a State or city . . . from expressing a preference for normal childbirth. . . .").

15. *Tileston v. Ullman*, 129 Conn. 84, 26 A.2d 582 (1942), appeal dismissed, 318 U.S. 44 (1943)

16. Under this principle, a woman with an uncomplicated pregnancy who suffered a fatal embolus during delivery would likewise have no opportunity to challenge the statute, because no "case or controversy" would exist at her death. See Morris V: Two women in early 30's die in childbirth at Yale-New Haven. New Haven Register, August 25, 1989, p 1. The article describes two women in their early 30s, previously in good health, who died while giving birth—one from an amniotic fluid embolus, the other from an undiagnosed cardiac abnormality. "These were totally unforeseen and unpreventable," a hospital spokesman is quoted as saying. If these women had sought abortions instead and were denied, no court has recognized that women could challenge abortion statutes based on the state's imposition of this risk of death. This is particularly remarkable in light of the rhetoric about the "fetal right to life" and the Supreme Court's recognition of the state's compelling interest in fetal life. "There is no comparable compelling state interest in women's lives."

17. Mohr (1978), pp 257–258. It is interesting to note the way antiabortion advocates distort Mohr's findings. In the *Webster* amicus brief filed by the U.S. Justice Department, the authors state, "The tenor and contemporaneous understanding of the antiabortion laws enacted from the mid-Nineteenth Century up to the time of the decision in *Roe v. Wade* leaves little doubt that they were directed not only at protecting maternal health, but also at what was widely viewed as a moral evil comprehending the destruction of actual or nascent human life. See J. Mohr, *Abortion in America* (1978)." Brief for the United States as amicus curiae supporting appellants, *Webster v. Reproductive Health Services*, 109 S.Ct. 3040 (1989).

Arguing that antiabortion laws were enacted at any period in history for the purposes of "protecting maternal health" is a laughable contention. This is particularly true for the twentieth century, but it is equally true of the nineteenth century, when "medical findings" were used to provide justifications for men's control over women's reproductive processes—a dynamic that continues today in the use of scientific material for the justification of ideological and political arguments. See brief amicus curiae of 167 distinguished scientists and physicians, *Webster v. Reproductive Health Services*, 109 S.Ct. 3040 (1989). Mere "rationalizations" ("for women's own good") disguise profoundly oppressive policies destructive of women's life, health and general well-being.

18. *Carey v. Population Services International*, 431 U.S. 678 (1977)

19. Morgan RG: *Roe v. Wade* and the lesson of pre-*Roe* case law. Michigan Law Review 77:1724–1748, 1979

20. *Loving v. Virginia*, 388 U.S. 1 (1967); *Skinner v. Oklahoma*, 316 U.S. 535 (1942); *Eisenstadt v. Baird, Prince v. Massachusetts*, 321 U.S. 158 (1944); *Pierce v. Society of Sisters*, 268 U.S. 510 (1925); *Meyer v. Nebraska*, 262 U.S. 390 (1923)

21. Some have challenged this view: Thomson JJ: A defense of abortion, in The Rights and Wrongs of Abortion. Edited by Cohen M, Nagel T, Scanlon T. Princeton, NJ, Princeton University Press, 1974. MacKinnon CA: Feminism Unmodified. Cambridge, MA, Harvard University Press, 1987, pp 93–102. MacKinnon CA: Towards a Feminist Theory of the State. Cambridge, MA, Harvard University Press, 1989, pp 184–194.

22. Rosenblum VG, Marzen TJ: Strategies for reversing *Roe v. Wade* through the courts, in Abortion and the Constitution: Reversing *Roe v. Wade* Through the Courts. Edited by Horan DJ, Grant ER, Cunningham PC. Washington, DC, Georgetown University Press, 1987, pp 195–214

23. Medically, this rationale is nonsensical in its attempt to create a medical "logic" for restriction of second-trimester abortion. According to the history of the *Roe* opinion, this "compelling point" was added to induce Chief Justice Warren Burger to join the opinion. Blackmun originally drafted the opinion to prohibit states from placing any significant restrictions on abortion before the point of viability; however, Burger balked at signing on to the opinion unless some provision was made for restrictions earlier in pregnancy. To get Burger's vote, Blackmun provided the additional "compelling point," which he justified as a state interest in protecting maternal health. As such, it is yet another example of how restrictions are placed on women's access to abortion (or contraception) with the paternalistic excuse that it is "for women's own good." This appears to be a dynamic common to both nineteenth- and twentieth-century abortion legislation and jurisprudence in which a thin rationalization varnishes motivations of power and control—in this case, male control over women's sexual and reproductive functions.

24. *Planned Parenthood of Central Missouri v. Danforth*, 428 U.S. 52 (1976)

25. *Planned Parenthood Assn. of Kansas City v. Ashcroft*, 462 U.S. 476 (1983); *Akron v. Akron Center for Reproductive Health*, 462 U.S. 416 (1983); *H.L. v. Matheson*, 450 U.S. 398 (1981); *Bellotti v. Baird (II)*, 443 U.S. 622 (1979); *Planned Parenthood of Central Missouri v. Danforth*, 428 U.S. 52 (1976)

It is difficult to know how carrying a pregnancy to term is in the "best interest" of any minor who seeks an abortion. The Supreme Court's opinions on teenage sexuality are contradictory. In *Michael M. v. Sonoma County Superior Court*, 450 U.S. 464 (1981), the court upheld a California statute that made men of all ages criminally liable for the act of sexual intercourse with a female younger than 18 years. In this opinion, Justice Rehnquist seemed to have no difficulty understanding what was at stake for young women. In writing for the majority, Rehnquist stated, "We need not be medical doctors to discern that young men and young women are not similarly situated with respect to the problems and the risks of sexual intercourse. Only women may become pregnant, and they suffer disproportionately the profound physical, emotional, and psychological consequences of sexual activity. The statute at issue here protects women from sexual intercourse at an age when those consequences are particularly severe." Despite Rehnquist's admonition that the burdens of unwanted pregnancy are disproportionately placed on women, Rehnquist would be unlikely to recognize that laws restricting abortion or contraception constitute sex discrimination under the Equal Protection Clause. The "logic" of law related to teenage sexuality is subtly misogynistic. For example, statutory rape laws assume that all minor females are unable to give proper consent to the act of intercourse (a questionable and paternalistic assertion), yet the argument that pregnancy per se is evidence of the commission of statutory rape and that an adolescent has an even greater claim to access to abortion is never entertained. Moreover, it never seems to be asked whether coercing a child to carry a pregnancy to term against her will constitutes child abuse. I have observed parents of unmarried minors refuse permission for an abortion for the stated reason that this was "punishment" for the child's sexual activity.

26. *Akron v. Akron Center for Reproductive Health*, 462 U.S. 416, 431 (1983)

27. *Planned Parenthood Assn. of Kansas City v. Ashcroft*, 462 U.S. 476 (1983); *Planned Parenthood of Missouri v. Danforth*, 428 U.S. 52 (1976); *Connecticut v. Menillo*, 423 U.S. 9 (1975); *Roe v. Wade*, 410 U.S. 113, 163–164 (1973)

28. The Supreme Court declared hospitalization requirements for all second-trimester abortions to be unconstitutional: *Doe v. Bolton*, 410 U.S. 179 (1973); *Akron v. Akron Center for Reproductive Health*, 462 U.S. 416 (1983); *Planned Parenthood of Kansas City, Mo., Inc. v. Ashcroft*, 462 U.S. 476 (1983).

29. *Roe v. Wade*, 410 U.S. 113 (1973). The Supreme Court's logic in restricting postviability abortions contains an internal contradiction. Viability is defined as the point at which a fetus is capable of meaningful life outside the uterus, albeit with artificial aid, yet the Court forbids the termination of gestation based on a stated affirmation of the fetus's supposed capacity for independent life. Thus the "logic" is that women can be forced to gestate a fetus based on the presumption that the fetus can live independently.

30. *Planned Parenthood Assn. of Kansas City v. Ashcroft*, 462 U.S. 506 (1983) (upheld the two-physician requirement)

31. *Thornburgh v. ACOG*, 476 U.S. 747, 759 (1986)

32. *Thornburgh v. ACOG*, 476 U.S. 747 (1986) (invalidated the Pennsylvania informed-consent provision); *Akron v. Akron Center for Reproductive Health*, 462 U.S. 416 (1983) (invalidated the *Akron* informed-consent ordinance); *Planned Parenthood of Central Missouri v. Danforth*, 428 U.S. 52 (1976) (upheld the reasonable-informed-consent requirement).

It is likely that the Rehnquist Court would reverse the Court's previous stance on informed-consent provisions. This is suggested in the dissent of Justices Rehnquist, White, and O'Connor in *Akron*, where they voted to uphold the same informed-consent provision that the majority struck down as unconstitutional. This provision required physicians to inform a woman that "the unborn child is a human life from the moment of conception," to inform her of the estimated gestational age of the pregnancy, and to provide detailed physiological information about fetal development (brain and heart function, sensitivity to pain, etc.) among other provisions. Physicians were also compelled by the *Akron* ordinance to inform a woman that "abortion is a major surgical procedure which can result in serious complications, including hemorrhage, perforated uterus, infection, menstrual disturbances, sterility and miscarriage and prematurity in subsequent pregnancies."

33. *Bigelow v. Virginia*, 421 U.S. 809 (1975)

34. *Akron v. Akron Center for Reproductive Health*, 462 U.S. 416 (1983)

35. *Doe v. Bolton*, 410 U.S. 179 (1973)

36. *Maher v. Roe*, 432 U.S. 464 (1977) (the Court upheld a Connecticut regulation limiting Medicaid reimbursement to "medically necessary" abortions only, despite state funding of childbirth expenses, on the grounds that the state may make a policy choice favoring "normal" childbirth over abortion); *Poelker v. Doe*, 432 U.S. 519 (1977) (upheld a city's refusal to provide publicly financed hospital services for "nontherapeutic" abortions while providing publicly financed hospital services for "normal" childbirth); *Beal v. Doe*, 432 U.S. 438 (1977) (upheld a Pennsylvania re-

striction on use of Medicaid funds for abortion, which barred payment except for those deemed "medically necessary"); *Williams v. Zbaraz*, 448 U.S. 358 (1980) (upheld an Illinois statute prohibiting use of state funds for abortion except when necessary to preserve the life of the woman undergoing the abortion); *Harris v. McRae*, 448 U.S. 297 (1980) (upheld the Hyde Amendment restricting the use of federal funds for abortion to those necessary to preserve the life of the woman undergoing the abortion).

37. The Hyde Amendment and legislation similar to the Hyde Amendment contain the underlying assumption that women control sex. In establishing an exception for rape or incest, it is otherwise assumed that all other acts of sexual intercourse leading to impregnation are voluntary or desired by a woman. For a critique of this view, see MacKinnon CA: Feminism Unmodified. Cambridge, MA, Harvard University Press, 1987, pp 93–1021; MacKinnon CA: Toward a Feminist Theory of the State. Cambridge, MA, Harvard University Press, 1989, pp 184–194. MacKinnon argues that women do not control sexual access to their bodies in any meaningful sense under conditions of sexual inequality.

38. Justice Brennan's dissent in *Harris v. McRae*, 448 U.S. 297, 338 (1980)

39. Justice Marshall's dissent in *Harris v. McRae*, 448 U.S. 297, 338 (1980)

40. *Akron v. Akron Center for Reproductive Health*, 462 U.S. 416, 419, n.1 (1983)

41. Although the Supreme Court does not explicitly call this new standard *rational-basis review*, the "permissibly furthers" standard essentially represents a lower standard of review. This is consistent with views previously expressed by Justices Rehnquist, White, and O'Connor. See *Roe v. Wade*, 410 U.S. 170, 173 (1973) (Rehnquist states that the "rational relation" test is appropriate for judicial review of abortion legislation), and *Thornburgh v. ACOG*, 476 U.S. 747, 828 (1986) (Justices O'Connor, Rehnquist, and White found that rational-basis review is appropriate for judicial review of abortion legislation that does not involve an absolute or severe obstacle to women's abortion decisions).

42. 462 U.S. 416, 445 (1983)

43. Human Life Center: The pill and IUD: abortive? Collegeville, MN, St. John's University, distributed by state chapters of the National Right to Life Committee. The pamphlet states: "in Stedman's 1976 edition, conception is defined as 'implantation of the blastocyst'—a week after fertilization. A mistake? Hardly. Officials of the American College of Obstetrics and Gynecology, officials in. . . . HEW (including FDA) and the U.S. Supreme Court, and others are trying to change the meaning of the word 'conception.' They now define it as the event and time of implantation of nidation . . . and they tell us that is when life begins."

44. The definition of life contained in the Illinois statutes is similar to that contained in the Missouri preamble in *Webster*. See 1987 Illinois Rev. Statues, Chap. 38, par. 81-21 through 81-22.

45. There is a great irony here: The assertion contained in the plurality opinion as well as Justice Scalia's broad assertion that the issues addressed in *Webster* are best left to politics are controverted by the plurality's own agreement that the state's interest in potential life does not simply begin at viability. Obviously, the Supreme Court's assertions of where the interests lie, and where they begin and end, are not part of the process of leaving it to the democratic process.

46. Justice Blackmun citing *West Virginia Board of Education v. Barrette*, 319 U.S. 624, 638 (1943) in *Webster v. Reproductive Health Services*, 109 S.Ct. 3040, 3077 n.11 (1989)

47. Wilkerson I: Missouri after the abortion ruling: both sides form their battle lines. New York Times, July 9, 1989, p 19. It is remarkable that the 1986 statute at issue in *Webster* passed with little legislative opposition: The statute passed 119 to

36 in the Missouri House and 23 to 5 in the Senate. This suggests that opposition to more severe restrictions may not be forthcoming in the Missouri legislature.

48. Wilkerson (1989)

49. These cases present a direct opportunity for the Supreme Court to overrule *Roe* either implicitly or explicitly. All of the cases involve state legislation creating obstacles to women's access to abortion during the first trimester. They include *Turnock v. Ragsdale*, No. 88-790 (an Illinois statute requires private abortion clinics to meet standards similar to those required of operating rooms in full-scale hospitals); *Hodgson v. Minnesota*, No. 88-1125, No. 88-1309 (a Minnesota statute requires notification of both parents before a teenage girl may undergo an abortion, even in situations of incest, divorce, or parental desertion); and *Ohio v. Akron Center for Reproductive Health*, No. 88-805 (an Ohio statute requires notification of at least one parent before a teenage girl may undergo an abortion). The parental notification statutes of Ohio and Minnesota contain provisions for a judicial bypass.

50. See Rehnquist's dissent in *Carey v. Population Services International*, 431 U.S. 678 (1977).

51. Dissenting in *Roe v. Wade* (1973), Rehnquist voiced skepticism about a constitutional right to privacy and argued that rationality review provided sufficient protection for judicial review of first-trimester regulations. He stated that he found the Supreme Court's trimester analysis inappropriate for the court and declared this function to be more properly that of the legislature. In addition, Rehnquist remarkably opened his comments on the case by stating that Jane Roe's suit was hypothetical because more than 9 months had elapsed since Roe originally filed her complaint and there was thus no longer a "case or controversy."

52. *Planned Parenthood v. Danforth*, 428 U.S. 52, 92 (1976); *Colautti v. Franklin*, 439 U.S. 379, 401 (1979); *Akron v. Akron Center for Reproductive Health*, 462 U.S. 416, 460 (1983); *Belotti v. Baird*, 443 U.S. 622, 656 (1979)

53. 1987 Illinois Revised Statutes, Chap. 38, par. 81-22, Sec. 2(7) (describes *abortifacient* as "any instrument, medicine, drug . . . which is known to cause fetal death when employed in the usual and customary use . . . whether or not the fetus is known to exist when such substance or device is employed"); Chap. 38, par. 81-31, Sec. 11(3) (declares it to be a Class C misdemeanor for a physician who prescribes an abortifacient to fail to inform the person for whom it is prescribed that the drug or instrument is an abortifacient).

54. See Dr. and Mrs. Wilke JC: Abortion: Questions and Answers. Cincinnati, OH, Hayes, 1988, p 231

55. Cited in Merton AH: Enemies of Choice. Boston, MA, Beacon, 1981, p 220

56. My personal files

57. See, e.g., Dr. and Mrs. Wilke JC: Abortion: Questions & Answers. Cincinnati, OH, Hayes, 1985, p 16 ("We don't know of a single pro-life or pro-abortion leader, or church leader, or congressman, or state representative who would want [women to be punished]. The mother is the second victim. . . . No, women would not be punished under a Human Life Amendment. Would the abortionist? Yes, he or she is the killer who took the money and did the abortion. The abortionist deserves punishment and would, in all probability, be punished, as in years past.")

58. Justice Blackmun's dissent in *Webster v. Reproductive Services*, 109 S.Ct. 3040, 3079 (1989)

Chapter 5

Values, Gender, and the Abortion Question: A Feminist Perspective

Lynn T. Shepler, M.D.

The gender bias that underlies the values and assumptions that shape abortion decisions is rarely scrutinized. Virginia Woolfe wrote in *A Room of One's Own*, "It is obvious that the values of women differ very often from the values which have been made by the other sex." Yet, she added, "it is the masculine values that prevail."[1]

It may not be obvious that men and women hold different values or reason differently regarding moral questions. Gender differences in moral reasoning have been demonstrated in the work of Carol Gilligan as well as that of Jean Piaget. However, the observed sexual differences in moral reasoning may not represent any inherent difference between the sexes, but simply the adaptations of a subordinate class under conditions of sexual inequality.[2]

The nature of this bias could be characterized as having five traits: 1) the valuation of men's experience over that of women's; 2) the failure to value women's health and well-being, including women's capacity for sexual expression as a positive moral good; 3) the overvaluation of a morality that is abstract and rule-bound—that is, "principled," as contrasted with contextual moral systems; 4) an invocation of tradition that ignores the patriarchal and misogynistic elements of historical practices; and 5) the antiwoman and antisexual ideology that has shaped Christian teaching on abortion and contraception.

Misogyny and the Devaluation of Woman

The negative moral dimensions of misogyny have been slow to be recognized. "Feminism," argued theologian Beverly Wildung Harrison, "is fundamentally a moral claim. . . . Many religious ethicists, moral theologians, and moral philosophers, mostly male, have discussed the morality of abortion, or of social policy relating to abortion, without reference to contemporary scholarly evidence that the disvaluation of women is deeply embedded in Western culture and constitutes an unacceptable moral heritage that requires correction."[3] The devaluation of women's experience and moral capacity is evident in the U.S. Supreme Court *Roe v. Wade* (1973) decision. Justice Harry Blackmun may be well-meaning, but he limits his inquiry on abortion to the views of men: "in this opinion [we] place some emphasis upon . . . what history reveals about man's attitudes towards the abortion procedure over the centuries."[4] At no turn of his lengthy discussion on the historical perspective of abortion does Blackmun present the view of a woman. Rather, the views of no fewer than 50 men are presented and discussed in some detail, as well as the views on abortion held by American medical and legal organizations dominated by men.

The Supreme Court has been silent on the question of the constitutional implications of a state's imposition of the risks of death or disability associated with childbirth. Concern for the physical well-being of women has never been a prominent focus of the modern jurisprudence on reproduction, which critics argue is more obsessed with physician rights and the nature of a state's intrusion on sexual relations. The Supreme Court identifies *maternal health* not as a right or interest of an individual woman but as an interest of the state. Maternal health is thus the rationalization permitting the state to regulate or restrict women's access to abortion. This is similar to the nineteenth-century rubric of "for her own good," which was used to justify a panoply of laws restricting women's movement in society.

The fleeting presence of the "state's compelling interest in maternal health" in the cases after *Roe v. Wade* and the rapidity with which it was eclipsed by the "state's interest in potential life" in subsequent cases reveals it to have been little more than a rationale for upholding abortion regulations. There is no mention of the risks attendant to childbirth, labor, and delivery other than for the medically specious purpose of calculating at what point regulation of second-trimester abortions is permissible.[5]

The misogyny that underlies the movement to enact cruel public policies on issues related to women's sexuality and reproductive functions is rarely acknowledged and may be seen as simply a side effect of a morally principled position of self-induced harm by women. We must ask what underlies the willingness to impose physical discomfort and pain on women—particularly in a society in which women are exposed to the constant threat of physical and sexual violence from strangers, husbands, lovers, and fathers. The perception that conception is voluntary or careless is often inaccurate. Studies indicate that unprotected sexual intercourse is forced on strangers, wives, lovers, and daughters under the threat or reality of physical, emotional, or financial abuse. If *Roe v. Wade* is reversed, women will likely die or may be maimed or mutilated. Such an outcome may be, on some level, the point.

U.S. political leaders evidence a profound indifference to women's health and well-being. Two presidential administrations and the Republican party have declared themselves in support of a constitutional amendment declaring that life should be protected from the moment of conception and of the reversal of *Roe v. Wade*. There have been no proposals to ease burdens on women or to support procreational choice with increased funding of contraceptive research or distribution. Two presidential administrations have applied an abortion litmus test for appointments to high-level administrative positions in the Department of Health and Human Services, provoking an outcry within the scientific community.[6] Particularly significant, given the paucity of research funds, is the fact that millions of dollars in government research funds have been channeled to Roman Catholic universities for research in techniques of natural family planning, a little-used and ineffective form of fertility control.[7]

Harrison argued that there is a "serious need to weigh the abortion controversy in a moral context which both affirms and advocates women's well-being. . . . Equally urgent is that more women come to appreciate that the considerable power of feminism in the lives of contemporary women is rooted not, as some have claimed, in women's growing selfishness, preoccupation with self, or even narcissism but in women's growing self-respect."[8]

Women are also devalued as sexual beings. Proponents of the recriminalization of abortion are also often equally opposed to contraception. Harrison stated, "In our Western biomedical, theological, and moral traditions, women consistently have been cast as passive vessels through which the power of male generation flows."[9] Sexuality, in the view of many conservatives, is not a form of intimacy and personal expression but a biological function for procreation. Within this framework, childbearing is not a woman's informed choice but her sole function.

Although the idea of procreational choice is new in Western society, it is essential for women's well-being. It should therefore be viewed as a positive and moral good rather than as simply a pragmatic compromise of moral principles. Sex-negative ideology prevalent during the Middle Ages still pervades Christian doctrine. Despite opposition to abortion from many Christian faiths, the Bible contains no specific injunction against abortion.

Abortion ethics often reflect underlying assumptions about the nature of women's labor, specifically women's reproductive labor. Some critics of the *Roe v. Wade* opinion have argued that abortion rights are more correctly grounded in notions of free labor and physical integrity than on an implicit constitutional right of privacy.[10] That women's domestic or reproductive labor has rarely been viewed or valued as anything other than natural goes some distance in explaining why no legal discourse has arisen to provide constitutional limits on state coercion of women's reproductive labor.

In American jurisprudence and historical tradition, the constitutional value of free labor is expressed in the Thirteen Amendment of the U.S. Constitution: "Neither slavery nor involuntary servitude except as a punishment for crime thereof the party shall have been duly convicted, shall exist within the United States, or any place subject to their jurisdiction." *Involuntary servitude* has been defined by the Supreme Court as "a condition of enforced compulsory service of one to another."[11] There can be no question that pregnancy, compelled by law, is a condition of enforced compulsory service of one to another, whether the women is laboring involuntarily for the fetus or for the production of a fetus for her husband or the state.

Although the Thirteenth Amendment has been applied to protect the labor of white men—going so far as to protect delinquent fathers against "seek-work" orders in child-support cases—the amendment has never been interpreted by the courts to apply to the sexual or reproductive labor of women.[12] Exploitation of women's reproductive labor was a necessary feature of American plantation slavery, in which rape and forced maternity resulted in the "natural" increase of the African slave population.[13] Female slaves were valued for their fertility, and the products of women's reproductive labor—children—were sold or used, in turn, by plantation owners to generate the economic wealth of the plantation.[14] In legal tradition, the injuries uniquely experienced by women under slavery and the value of women's free labor have been recognized by the courts only insofar as women's experience and labor approximate men's. Thus Thirteenth Amendment arguments for abortion rights have been repeatedly rejected by the courts, who, it seems, eschew recognition of pregnancy and childbirth as labor, preferring to cast childbearing in its more abstract dimensions. Choice, the Supreme Court tells us, is the nature of the abortion right protected by the constitutional right of privacy. The privacy doctrine thus imperceptibly sustains the invisible quality of women's reproductive labor, which is currently unrecognized as labor per se in the social sphere and continues to be unrecognized as labor for the purposes of constitutional protections.

Epistemology and the Moral Capacity of Woman

Implicit in the debate about state regulation of abortion is an underlying assumption about the moral incapacity of women. Harrison noted, "Nothing makes clearer how little women count as full, valued persons or as competent moral agents" than the proposals that make "the state the controller of procreation."[15] The debate about a woman's moral capacity is as old as Aristotle and Hippocrates. It was discussed by Freud and developed in the work of feminist philosophers and theologians during the last decade.[16] Before the research of Carol Gilligan, Lawrence Kohlberg advanced the theory that only males achieved the highest rung of moral development, which he defined as the ability to apply abstract principles of moral justice to situations of social conflict. Gilligan argues that it is not that women are any less able to reason about moral issues but that women's values and the way in which women define themselves in relation to the world differ from men's.

Problems of moral conflict may be resolved differently depending on gender, according to Gilligan. Boys and men are more likely to resolve competing moral claims through the application of abstract principles. Resolution of moral conflict in girls and women appears to be more a function of social context and existing human relations within a conflict than an application of principles.

Applying these findings to the abortion question, abortion ethics could be argued to be masculinist where the answer to a question about abortion is seen to hinge on the abstract proposition of whether a clump of cells is indeed human.[17] If the clump of cells is deemed human, the inquiry ends. This type of analysis is contained in Justice Blackmun's reasoning in *Roe v. Wade*: A woman's right to abortion ends with the recognition of fetal personhood. Within this type of analysis, fetal personhood takes absolute priority over other constitutional values or rights of others; the social context is irrelevant.[18] Thus in a traditional, masculinist-based epistemology of abortion, the question about abortion rights may indeed be short.

Feminist philosophers and legal scholars describe how gendered notions of the self construct discussion.[19] Western thought constructs the self as separate, autonomous, and rational and creates dichotomies in which underlying metaphors of gender are present in the opposing elements; male/female, mind/body, reason/emotion, law/desire, civilization/nature, order/chaos, ad infinitum. The mind/body dualism provides the structure for the Supreme Court discourse on therapeutic versus nontherapeutic abortions and medically necessary versus medically unnecessary abortions. Even in the twentieth century, the mind may be the realm of the masculine—a realm in which women do not participate. Woman, in essence, is body, her control recognized where it is sanctioned by medicine and only where life itself is at stake.

Therapeutic versus nontherapeutic abortion? Certainly for every woman who seeks an abortion to terminate an unwanted pregnancy, an abortion is therapeutic or medically necessary. Abortion is medically necessary for every woman so desperate as to risk her life in ending that pregnancy. In the modern law of abortion, the well-being of woman counts only in terms of her physical state, and then little at all.[20] The metaphors of gender discovered in epistemologic dichotomies also underpin the cultural mythology that men are better able to distribute justice (or to decide about abortion) based on their ability to be detached, rational, or objective, contrasted with the nature of women—irrational, emotionally labile, and swayed by contextuality.

The rhetoric of political liberalism also contains metaphors of gender and assumptions based on a gendered self. The polity is an association of separate, autonomous, rational individuals; values of rights and individuality are asserted over values of community and notions of obligation; a laissez-faire posture is preferred to social or economic regulation; choice, reflecting the values of freedom and liberty, is valued over equality. Public discourse on procreational choice is poorly served by the rhetoric of political liberalism, in which abortion easily comes to take on the meaning of choice for choice's sake. Privacy, grounded in liberalism's value of laissez-faire state nonintervention, which is in turn premised on a gendered self that is autonomous and separate, fails to capture the nature of procreational relations. Indication that procreational choice is a substantive moral good, and not simply an extension of political liberalism's choice run amok, is absent from liberalism's rhetoric, which eschews recognition of the dependent and profoundly socially based nature of procreational relations. Privacy, as a value on which to ground women's procreational choice, has little to recommend it as a moral theory. Women's basic needs and desires to exercise control over their reproductive functions should be fostered by the state as a public social good available to all women—not the exercise of a private choice characterized as a matter of state indifference, available to only some.[21]

Invoking Tradition: Whose?

The constitutional foundation for reproductive rights is one of the most hotly debated legal issues of modern times. One of the critical inquiries in the constitutional debate is the following: Is abortion a right "so rooted in the traditions and conscience of our people as to be ranked fundamental"?[22] The awkwardness of the question is itself striking, although the question appears structured to answer itself. Could anyone argue with assurance that a man's right to a kidney transplant or femoral-popliteal bypass is rooted in the tradition and conscience of our people?

Although medical practice has changed, the general principle that an individual has a right to bodily security is as alive in modern times as it was during the time of its initial enunciation by political liberalism's early philosophers.[23] The modern question is, Will these principles be extended equally to women? The right to privacy as conceived by the Supreme Court begs that the question be asked. That the court has balked at granting women the same rights held by men is likely why both sides in the abortion conflict find the right articulated in *Roe v. Wade* to lack substance.[24]

The practice of abortion may qualify as a tradition if tradition is defined as a set of customs or practices transmitted from generation to generation, particularly when abortion is viewed in its eighteenth- and nineteenth-century context. It was the great power of this tradition—which was woman's—that male "regulars" relentlessly sought to root out from social practice.

The status of abortion in American common law also supports this view. In most states, abortion of an unquickened fetus was not considered a criminal act. In other states, such as Maryland or New York, abortion of a quick fetus was considered a misdemeanor. Abortion, as a social practice, was part of the fabric of early American life. Conservatives ignore women's culture. Citing the intention of the framers of the U.S. Constitution (which did not include racial or sexual equality), they turn a blind eye to the indifference to women of American constitutional tradition and the intense misogyny that fueled the enactment of antiabortion and contraception legislation during the nineteenth century.

Invoking religious tradition is equally problematic. Modern Christianity is tinged with the sex-negative, misogynistic ideology of early Christianity. Reproductive ethics in the context of a religious tradition that deifies males—led by a male hierarchy, often celibate—automatically raises questions about tradition's sensitivity to women and the oppressive function of religious tradition in maintaining patriarchal domination. Women's position in most religious tradition has been solely that of mother; childbearing is women's function rather than women's informed option. Invoking tradition often means invoking oppressive social and religious practices in contradiction to the constitutional guarantees that should be available to all citizens regardless of gender.

The Maternal-Fetal Conflict: Failure of the Moral and Scientific Imagination

Perhaps one of the most remarkable aspects of the abortion debate is that it is a debate. What does it mean, in a deeper and more serious sense, that twentieth-century scientific, legal, and political discourse pits a mother against a fetus?

Technically, the debate seems to be a conflict that could be solved or at least mitigated by the search for a safe, effective, reversible, and easy-to-use form of contraception. In the science-fiction world of reproductive technologies, other-worldly questions are asked about the making of test-tube babies, ex utero gestation, genetic engineering, and cloning of the self. Why, at the end of the twenty-first century, will we speak of the new reproductive technologies and not the new contraceptive technologies?

One answer is that science is not merely an abstract process but a social enterprise. Historically a vehicle for largely male scientific interests, science has had little time or interest in applying twentieth-century technology to the fertility-control problems of individual women. And when it seems that men or nations benefit as a result of women's disability, there is even less incentive to undertake the necessary investigations.

Investment in the development of contraception has effectively been staunched by conservative administrations. The current budget for the Contraceptive Development Branch at the National Institutes of Health scarcely exceeds $10 million. Since its founding in the 1960s when the U.S. Congress subsidized contraceptive development out of concern for population overgrowth, the budget of the Contraceptive Development Branch has been essentially unchanged.[25] Moreover, the orientation of the branch is not to serve the health care needs of individual women but to serve the population-control needs of governments. Under the last three Republican administrations, appointment of the branch's administrators has been contingent on each candidate's view on abortion.[26]

It is not simply that science has failed to provide for the reproductive health care needs of women; scientific findings and technological breakthroughs are continually invoked to argue for women's subjugation to biological processes.[27] This is similar to the use of science during the nineteenth century when "scientific" evidence of women's natural inferiority was used to justify the exclusion of women from public life.

Toward a Feminist Ethic of Abortion

Women ethicists, theologians, and writers, including Harrison and Christine Overall, have begun to contemplate a feminist ethic of abortion.[28] Feminism's alienation from traditional notions of morality, in which questions of morality and ethics have been historically answered with misogynistic, sex-negative moralism, leaves the impression that reproductive ethics is "owned" by antiabortion advocates. Feminist and nonfeminist approaches to reproductive ethics diverge in their respective androcentric and gynocentric perspectives. The feminist perspective is grounded in women's experience and incorporates an awareness of women's historical oppression under patriarchy and a determination to end sexual inequality.[29]

Nonfeminist approaches to questions of reproductive ethics tend to center on the issue of abortion and the metaphysical topic of personhood. Overall noted, "There is . . . little discussion of the woman who is the co-creator and sole sustainer of the embryo/fetus, except as she is treated as a container or 'environment' for it."[30]

An ethic interested in women's well-being postulates a society in which women have true control over their sexual and reproductive powers. "Women have said again and again 'This body is my body!' and they have reason to feel angry, reason to feel that it has been shouting into the wind."[31] This includes not simply control over her body for reproductive purposes but also control of sexual exploitation and the sexual servicing of men. In the words of Catharine MacKinnon, it is notable that "the struggle for reproductive freedom has never included a woman's right to refuse sex."[32]

A feminist ethic would include the following elements, as delineated by Christine Overall, elements that are already ongoing demands by the women's movement:

1. Research into and development of safe, effective, reversible, low-cost contraceptive methods, and widespread distribution of birth planning information
2. A focus on abortion as a service for women, that is, the adequate provision of abortion clinics where the service is medically sound and easily available early in pregnancy
3. The direction of medical resources to discovering and reducing the causes of infertility
4. Examining and changing our attitudes toward and treatment of children, a process that would include the encouragement of general feelings of responsibility toward all children, the eradication of pronatalist pressures, and the questioning of the alleged importance of a genetic link to one's children
5. Withdrawal of any support for research into or implementation of technology that increases or contributes to preferences for male offspring
6. Promoting healthy pregnancies and joyous childbirth, financing paid maternity leave, and supporting all parents and caregivers in their efforts to provide the best for our children
7. Finally, most generally and most important, returning reproductive responsibility and power to women and enabling us to recognize and act on the real choices that must be made about the provision of reproductive services, support for research, and the regulation of new reproductive technology.[33]

The Role of Physicians

The issue of physician participation in the abortion decision is a product of the history of antiabortion legislation, which sought to drive out midwives and the tradition of women's self-help remedies. Progress in medicine also robbed women of the culture that supported women's intergenerationally transmitted methods of procreative control and support.

Strangely, although the Supreme Court opinion that upheld state legislation mandating that only *licensed physicians* perform abortions appears to be only a rational extension of modern licencing requirements for the protection of public health, this was one of the primary endpoints sought by the American Medical Association in its role as the driving force behind antiabortion legislations during the late 1800s. As a result, physicians are now the sole gatekeepers for women's access to a host of methods for fertility control. Our view of our twentieth-century role should be tempered by this historical understanding.

The doctrine of informed consent, based on the notions of bodily integrity and personal autonomy, is part of the tradition of twentieth-century medical practice.[34] These notions are values that permeate medical practice and are enshrined in political liberalism, the U.S. Constitution, and American constitutional law. John Locke, one of the founding fathers of political liberalism, was also a physician.

Procreational choice can and should be valued as a positive and moral good. Ethical principles that ground the doctrine of informed consent form the same ethical ground for a woman's decision whether to carry a pregnancy to term. It is not simply a matter of physical integrity but also a matter of personal self-expression: "We need to recognize that sexual self-determination is a right, and sexual pleasure is a foundational value that enhances human well-being and self-respect."[35]

Subtle distinctions about what is natural or desired shape abortion ethics in almost imperceptible ways. Unwanted conception, rather than abortion, is the "tragic" occurrence.[36] For some women, abortion is one of their first acts expressive of individual dignity and self-worth. Questions about physician involvement in abortion counseling are usually cast in terms of whether physicians may ethically and affirmatively counsel a woman to terminate her pregnancy. An equally legitimate question is, May physicians ethically withhold information on abortion or counsel against abortion in the context of a woman's deteriorating medical or psychological condition, or against her stated need? This question will be increasingly asked in our clinical practice if legislatures are permitted, by the courts and the electorate, to enact regulatory schemes restricting abortion.

We should not forget that it is not only our patients' access to reproductive health care that is threatened, but our own. Men and children, as well as women, have interests in protecting legal access to abortion. New antiabortion legislation will be effective only insofar as it can induce physicians to cease providing abortion care because of civil or criminal penalties, including the threat of loss of licensure. New abortion and contraceptive legislation is likely to conflict with our values and with our patients' values.

Ethical difficulties will be compounded whether we agree to comply with the law or refuse, compromising our liberty to practice medicine in the manner of its most-respected traditions.

Notes

1. Woolf V: A Room of One's Own. New York, Harcourt, Brace & World, 1929, p 76

2. MacKinnon CA: Towards a Feminist Theory of the State. Cambridge, MA, Harvard University Press, 1989, p 51. MacKinnon critiques Carol Gilligan's work on gender differences in moral reasoning. MacKinnon stated, "When difference means dominance as it does with gender, for women to affirm differences is to affirm the qualities and characteristics of powerlessness. Women may have an approach to moral reasoning, but it is an approach made both of what is and of what is not allowed to be . . . . Women are said to value care. Perhaps women value care because men have valued women according to the care they give."

3. Harrison BW: Our Right to Choose: Toward a New Ethic of Abortion. Boston, MA, Beacon, 1983, p 7

4. *Roe v. Wade*, 410 U.S. 113, 118 (1973)

5. This compelling point is calculated to be the point at which the mortality rate of abortion approaches that of childbirth.

6. Pro-choice? Get lost: antiabortion views are a must at Health and Human Services. Time, December 4, 1989; Koshland DE: The choosing of the NIH director. Science 246:981, 1989; Culliton BJ: Abortion: litmus test for NIH director. Science 246:27, 1989

7. Johnson JH, Reich J: The new politics of natural family planning. Fam Plann Perspect 18:277–282, 1986

8. Harrison (1983), pp 4, 48

9. Harrison (1983), p 10

10. Regan DH: Rewriting *Roe v. Wade*. Michigan Law Review 77:1569–1646, 1979. MacKinnon (1989) stated, "Even before *Roe v. Wade*, arguments for abortion under the rubric of feminism have rested upon the right to control one's own body, gender neutral. This argument has been appealing for the same reasons it is inadequate: socially, women's bodies have not been theirs; women have not controlled their meanings and destinies" (p 189).

11. *Hodges v. United States*, 203 U.S. 1, 16 (1906)

12. *Dimon v. Dimon*, 40 Cal. 2d 516, 254 P.2d 528 (1953); *Ex parte Todd*, 119 Cal. 57, 58; *Pollock v. Williams*, 322 U.S. 4, 18 (1944) (explaining the prohibitions of the Thirteenth Amendment as implemented by the Antipeonage Act: "congress has put it beyond debate that no indebtedness warrants a suspension of the right to be free from compulsory service . . . or make criminal sanctions available for holding unwilling persons to labor."); *Bailey v. Alabama*, 219 U.S., 240–241 (1910) (the Thirteenth Amendment was not intended to apply only to African slavery but was a "charter of universal civil freedom for all persons"); *Hodges v. United States*, 203 U.S. 1, 16 (1906).

Involuntary-servitude arguments have even been used to defend men against child-support orders requiring a divorced father to make a search for other employment to increase or to add to his limited income. *In Re Marriage of Dennis*, 117 Wis. 2d 249, 344 N.W. 2d 128 (1984) (where a concurring judge raised the issue that a seek-work order "raises questions of due process, equal protection, and involuntary servitude. . . .")

13. The exploitation of African women's reproductive functions was a significant factor in the development of southern plantation wealth and a well-described dimen-

sion of women's experience under slavery. Gutman HG: The Black Family in Slavery and Freedom, 1750–1925. New York, Random House, 1976; Gutman HG: Slavery and the Numbers Game. Urbana, IL, University of Illinois Press, 1975; Kolchin P: Unfree Labor: American Slavery and Russian Serfdom. Cambridge, MA, Harvard University Press, 1987; Lerner G: The Origins of Patriarchy. New York, Oxford University Press, 1986, pp 88–89; White D: Ar'n't I a Woman? Female Slaves in the Plantation South. New York, WW Norton, 1985. Reproductive exploitation of female slaves has been described in other systems of slavery throughout history: Gardner JF: Women in Roman Law and Society. Bloomington, IN, Indiana University Press, 1986; Bradley KR: The age at time of sale of female slaves. Arethusa 11:243–252, 1978

14. Alarm about low fertility rates by modern governments are similarly related to economic concerns, in addition to providing political hegemony through a large population. Herrnstein RJ: IQ and falling birth rates. The Atlantic 263 (May), 1989. Herrnstein associates American economic efficiency with fertility rates among educated women: "The competing ideals of [sexual] equality and efficiency create a dilemma of long standing. . . . The goal of efficient production competes with the goal of a more equal distribution of wealth." He concludes that "we ought to bear in mind that in not too many generations differential fertility could swamp the effect of anything else we may do about our economic standing in the world." Thus the state has usurped the position of the plantation owner in the modern exploitation of women's reproductive capacities.

15. Harrison (1983), p 35

16. Gilligan C: In a Different Voice: Psychological Theory and Women's Development. Cambridge, MA, Harvard University Press, 1982; Flax J: Political philosophy and the patriarchal unconscious: a psychoanalytic perspective on epistemology and metaphysics, in Discovering Reality: Feminist Perspectives on Epistemology, Metaphysics, Methodology and Philosophy of Science. Edited by Harding S, Hintikka MB. Boston, MA, D Reidel, 1983, pp 245–281; Harding S: The Science Question in Feminism. Ithaca, NY, Cornell University Press, 1986; Harrison (1983)

17. I use the term *masculinist* to refer to the male gender. I wish to imply that I believe all men or women conform to gender stereotypes; there are discernable traits or characteristics that can be attributed to gender.

18. Blackmun's reasoning is flawed in his assumption that abortion rights are abrogated when fetal personhood is recognized. He wrongly assumes the existence of a background common law whereby a state may coerce individuals to provide aid to others involuntarily. Given present law on the duty to aid, a woman still could not be compelled to provide her body for the gestation of another human being—even when that human being may not survive as a result. For example, a man may not be coerced to donate his kidney or bone marrow to his dying child, even when he is the only living donor and the child's survival could be guaranteed as a result of the transplant. See Regan (1979); Thomson JJ: A defense of abortion, in The Rights and Wrongs of Abortion. Edited by Cohen M, Nagel T, Scanlon T. Princeton, NJ, Princeton University Press, 1974.

19. Harding S, O'Barr JF (eds): Sex and Scientific Inquiry. Chicago, IL, University of Chicago Press, 1987; Harding S, Hintikka MB (eds): Discovering Reality: Feminist Perspectives on Epistemology, Metaphysics, Methodology, and Philosophy of Science, Boston, MA, D Reidel, 1983; West R: Jurisprudence and gender. University of Chicago Law Review 55:1, 1988. See, in particular, Flax J: Political philosophy and the patriarchal unconscious: a psychoanalytic perspective on epistemology and metaphysics, in Harding and Hintikka (1983), pp 245–281

20. *Harris v. McRae*, 448 U.S. 297 (1980), in which the Supreme Court upheld the Hyde Amendment, which permits states to refuse Medicaid coverage for "med-

ically necessary" abortions, even when continuing the pregnancy may result in severe permanent damage to the woman's health.

21. Harrison (1983), pp 54–55

22. In deciding whether an interest should be deemed a "fundamental right," the Supreme Court has indicated that an interest will be deemed to be constitutionally fundamental if it is "implicit in the concept of ordered liberty" or "deeply rooted in this Nation's history and tradition." *Palko v. Connecticut*, 302 U.S. 319, 325 (1937); *Moore v. East Cleveland*, 431 U.S. 494, 503 (1977). The question of historical tradition is therefore extremely important and bears on the question of what degree of constitutional protections will be afforded women's right to abortion.

23. It is of interest that these principles regarding the inviolate nature of the individual's right to bodily security were elaborated by John Locke, a physician, and one of the founders of liberalism.

24. Ely J: The wages of crying wolf: a comment on *Roe v. Wade*. Yale Law Journal 82:920, 1973; Epstein R: Substantive due process by any other name: the abortion cases. Supreme Court Review, 1973, p 159; Regan (1979)

25. The National Institutes of Health are also forbidden, through limits placed on the agency by congressional legislation, to investigate any form of contraception that is abortifacient in nature. Under current agency guidelines, the IUD and low-dose oral contraceptives could not have been developed.

26. Hilts PJ: Does anybody want to lead N.I.H. if job lasts only till next election? New York Times, September 8, 1989, p A12. (The article suggests that the removal of the previous director of the NIH, Dr. James B. Wyngaarden, may have been a function of his previous statement that women should be allowed to choose abortion in case of an unwanted pregnancy.) Selection of the current secretary of Health and Human Services, Dr. Louis Sullivan, also appeared contingent on his publicly stated views on abortion.

27. Wilke Dr & Mrs JC: Abortion: Questions and Answers. Cincinnati, OH, Hayes, 1988, p v. "[A] flood of new scientific information, particularly the explosion of detailed information about the other patient (the tiny one) through recent technology and modern research, reshapes our answers [on abortion]. . . . Many new facts have been confirmed by scientific studies."

28. Harrison (1983); Overall C: Reproductive ethics: feminist and nonfeminist approaches. Canadian Journal of Women and the Law 1:271–278, 1986; Overall C: Ethics and Human Reproduction: A Feminist Analysis. Boston, MA, Allen & Unwin, 1987

29. Overall (1986), pp 271–272

30. Overall (1986), pp 271, 273

31. Thomson JJ: A defense of abortion, in The Rights and Wrongs of Abortion. Edited by Cohen M, Nagel T, Scanlon T. Princeton, NJ, Princeton University Press, 1974.

32. MacKinnon (1989), p 188

33. Overall (1986), pp 277–278

34. Brief of the American Medical Association, American Academy of Child and Adolescent Psychiatry, American Academy of Pediatrics, American College of Obstetricians and Gynecologists, American Fertility Society, American Medical Women's Association, American Psychiatric Association, and American Society of Human Genetics as amici curiae in support of appellees. *Webster v. Reproductive Health Services*, 109 S. Ct. 3040 (1989)

35. Harrison (1983), p 39

36. See Chapter 14: "We must elicit and interpret the patient's preferences and try to understand the life circumstances that led to the tragic decision to terminate a pregnancy."

Chapter 6

Contraception: Use and Failure

Elisabeth C. Small, M.D.

The Human Population: Demographic, Economic, and Cultural Factors

Demography and Its Implications

Any discussion of fertility control entails considerations of a global and personal nature. At about 2% per year, population growth now is at the highest rate in humankind's experience. The world is adding nearly 80 million people per year, about as many as the population of the eighth-largest country, Bangladesh (Freedman and Berelson 1974). This growth rate is the difference between the birth rate and the death rate. Industrialization, technological development, and rapid scientific progress have led to a decrease in death rates, an increase in life expectancy, and a marked increase in the reproductive rate. Modern population growth is thought to be of crisis proportions because of the effect on the quality of life of individuals in developed and developing countries.

There is a disparity in the rate of population growth between developed and developing nations, with the most rapid rate in the less-developed areas. According to projections by the United Nations, more than 90% of the population increase anticipated by 2000 will be in the Third World, although a reduction in fertility had been anticipated. Some areas have actively supported programs of education and provision of birth control.

Where there is illiteracy, poverty, and a rural environment with poor health services, population control has fared poorly. The resultant social and economic problems are very serious.

The lack of effective fertility control is also associated with the global crisis of concentration of populations in the major cities of the world. Because core cities are the seats of industrial and economic growth, people flock to these areas in search of work, economic advantages, and a higher standard of living than is available in the rural periphery and in the slower-growing provincial cities and towns. Cities in the Third World and in developed countries are crowded and polluted to the limit (Vining 1985). The rapid growth in cities demands levels of housing, transportation, water, sanitation, and schools that strain the poorer countries as well as those that are more industrialized. Most governments spend disproportionate funds to meet these needs.

The conquest of nature and the control of death improves the quality of living mainly for a select population. Infants born to poverty-level mothers who do not practice effective fertility control are at greater risk of mortality and are more likely to be born under conditions of poor prenatal care; exposure to maternal illicit-drug use; exposure to acquired immunodeficiency syndrome (AIDS) and other infections; and prematurity, low birth weight, brain damage, and cardiac and other organ malformations. These infants require costly acute medical care and may require chronic lifetime maintenance. Projecting the American experience to the underdeveloped countries, one can predict the calamity resulting from reproductive growth in the face of an inadequate supporting environment for that growth (Brown 1987).

Cultural considerations involved in the attitudes toward fertility affect fertility rates. In developed countries, the trend has been generally downward. In contrast, the rate of increase in population in the less-developed countries spiraled from 1850 to 1960 because of a decrease in mortality and a sustained fertility rate. Since the 1960s, however, certain modernizing countries have made efforts to decelerate growth by strong family planning. Reduction of fertility is noted mainly in east Asia (Singapore, Taiwan, China, Hong Kong, and South Korea) and moderately in several small countries (Puerto Rico, Cuba, Brazil, Colombia, Venezuela, and Thailand), whereas much less reduction occurs in the Middle East. Tropical Africa has had no decline in birth rate (Keyfitz 1989).

Cultural Factors

The change from an agrarian to an industrialized economy has been coupled with changes in social and religious values. In an agrarian setting, children were an economic advantage and asset. In an industrial setting, children can be an economic drain on income and resources. The decline in traditional and religious authority released individuals from conformity to marital guidelines. Ethics of individuality and rationality predominate. Equal opportunities for education and the increasing status of equality for women open opportunities for career and employment that result in post-ponement of marriage. The increasing survival of children precludes having to procreate more. A consumer-oriented culture directed at maximizing personal gratification makes sharing and deprivation less appealing. Access to information and practice of birth-control methods further reduce the risk of pregnancy, without the imposition of celibacy.

Changes in the marital relationship affect fertility rates. Non-marriage has become more socially acceptable. In 1960, 29% of American women between the ages of 20 and 24 years had never been married. In 1978, 45% had never been married. There is a corresponding change in attitude about early marriage. Postponement of marriage until age 30 is often preferred by women who are occupied with work or career. In agrarian times, the earlier a woman married and could beget children, the more favorable she was to the economy: she reduced the cost of her maintenance to her nuclear family, and she enhanced the economic condition of her family by marrying and providing children as potential workers and as security in old age. For women in the industrial and postindustrial age, employment and children are not always compatible. Acceptance of cohabitation has allowed a period of time as a prelude to marriage, but it often means lower fertility because of its trial nature and its instability. In developed countries, such as Denmark, 25% of women between the ages of 18 and 25 years live with men to whom they are not married. In Sweden, 12% of couples between the ages of 16 and 70 years who are living together are not married.

Divorce may affect fertility rates. For a large U.S. population in which one in three marriages is expected to end in divorce, marriage "for life" is no longer a norm. With a high divorce rate, it is interesting that the re-marriage rate is also high. This suggests that the disenchantment may not necessarily be with the concept of marriage, but with the given spouse. The institution of marriage appears to have lost its sociological rationale in functional economic terms as a system whereby women offer babies and domestic services in exchange for the status and security of a man's income and occupation. In the United States, where more than 50% of the couples living together have both parties working to support the family, having fewer children facilitates the economic capability of the woman, which enhances the family income. Changes in marriage and family have a long-range impact on the declining population growth in industrialized countries. Those factors involved with the changing status of women are yet to be determined (Westoff 1978).

Sources of fertility limitation in preindustrialized populations were often associated with such marriage customs as late marriages, high numbers of permanently single individuals, and prohibition of remarriage for widows.

This limited many women from exposure to sexual contact and thus to reproductive risk. The prolongation of intervals between pregnancies, such as long and frequent episodes of breast-feeding, served as a natural method of birth control. Customs that forbade resumption of coitus for long periods after childbirth and forced frequent separation of spouses, such as seasonal migrations, also served as a barrier to fertility. Societies in Asia and Africa that encourage early marriage also support long interbirth periods by some of these practices. Modernization and contact with Western practices have had negative impacts on natural birth-control practices. Breast-feeding has decreased in some countries, such as South Korea, because of a high social value on milk-formula feeding (promoted through marketing of infant formulas). Since this change, a rise in fertility has been noted (Coale 1983). People must necessarily come to realize how their childbearing affects the future ecological stability of their country and the planet (Keyfitz 1989).

Contraception: History

The history of the birth-control movement in the United States dates to the early 1830s and was punctuated by colorful personalities—both proponents and antagonists of contraception. In 1831, Robert Dale Owen published the first American book on contraception describing the condom and the sponge, both of which were regarded as doubtfully effective. Owen proposed coitus interruptus as the preferred method. In 1832, Charles Knowlton suggested postcoital douching with various chemicals and herbals, and he placed responsibility for birth control on the female. Between 1858 and 1870, Edward Bliss Foote wrote books and pamphlets on contraception, supported use of the condom and cervical diaphragm, and presented indications for their use that included social, economic, medical, and eugenic factors. The vaginal diaphragm appeared in the 1880s in Holland, but it received little attention in the United States until the next century. By the early twentieth century, reproductive physiology was clarified and effective contraceptive techniques included not only condoms, cervical caps, and vaginal diaphragms, but also spermicides and newly developed intrauterine devices; however, without adequate education in contraceptive use and without access to this technology, the public had little awareness of the potential for fertility control.

Among the most significant opponents of birth control was Anthony Comstock. His efforts to combat artificial contraception resulted in the Comstock Act, signed by U.S. President Ulysses S. Grant on March 6,1873. This bill ordered that "No article, or thing, designed or intended, for the prevention of conception or notice of any kind in writing or print, giving information directly or indirectly, where or how, or of whom, or by what means either of the things before mentioned may be obtained or made, shall be carried in the mail." Comstock arranged to become the first special agent of the postmaster general to enforce this law. In this position, he zealously pursued convictions in such numbers as to boast that he had convicted enough persons to fill 61 coaches of a passenger train with 60 persons each. The Comstock Act influenced separate state governments to enact statutes that further prohibited giving information on contraception, prohibiting statements as to where such information was available, and even stating that mere possession of contraceptive materials was punishable. Contraception was associated with pornographic and obscene materials (Speert 1980).

The Comstock Act stood for nearly a century before it was finally repealed on January 8, 1971. Individual states subsequently began to repeal their laws restricting use of contraceptives.

The foremost proponent of fertility control was Margaret Higgins Sanger, who founded the first birth-control clinic. As a nurse, whose mother died of tuberculosis after bearing 11 children, Sanger made a career of the study and practice of contraception. In 1914, she published the magazine *Woman Rebel*, in which she first used the term *birth control*. Most of the issues of the magazine were banned by the post office. She was indicted and convicted of sending contraceptive information through the mail and sentenced to a prison term of 45 years. On the eve of her trial, she eloped to Europe. After 2 years, the indictment was lifted. After returning to the United States, she and her sister, Ethel Byrne, also a nurse, opened the first birth-control clinic in Brooklyn, New York, on October 16, 1916. This resulted in a 30-day jail sentence for Sanger, who was convicted for "public nuisance." Sanger went on to organize the National Birth Control League, which in 1942 became the Planned Parenthood Federation of America. With women from other countries, she formed the International Planned Parenthood Federation in 1952. Her willingness to accept public ridicule, and the legal and political consequences of her efforts to advocate and to gain endorsement of the birth-control movement, made her one of the most conspicuous leaders in the making of population-control policy. Sanger died in 1966 at the age of 82.

Religion plays a role in contraceptive practice. Of all of the major religions practiced in the United States, the Roman Catholic Church holds the most rigid stance against artificial contraception. A papal encyclical in 1968, stating that only the rhythm method was approved, has been associated with an extensive defection of Catholics from adherence to church dogma on birth control. It is estimated that two-thirds of Catholic women in the United States are using unapproved techniques and that, among women younger than 30, users are even more numerous. Some Catholic Latin American countries, such as Mexico, have not only accepted family planning programs but are also fairly active in their support, provided that in their educational efforts, periodic abstinence is also included and that no coercion is applied (Westhoff and Bumpass 1973).

From a federal government perspective, birth control as an issue began with the intent to aid developing countries with high birth rates and subsequently with concern with the American poor. Assistance to other countries soon brought attention to the rapidly increasing population among the poor minority sectors in the United States, and by 1961, the National Institutes of Health were assuming research responsibility for fertility studies and control, involving public hospitals and health departments in providing family-planning care. Agencies such as the National Center for Family Planning Service, the Office of Population Affairs, and the Commission on Population Growth and the American Future were involved in family-planning assistance to women with low incomes. The ideal goals of the commission were "to reduce fertility, to improve pregnancy outcome, to improve the health of children," and to recommend private and public financing to meet the cost of health care related to fertility. The expansive nature of the program was to include contraception; prenatal, obstetrical, and postpartum care; pediatric care for the first year of life; voluntary sterilization; termination of unwanted pregnancy; and treatment of infertility (Speert 1980). Currently, federal funding programs separate contraceptive research from family-planning services. Contraceptive-development research is performed under the auspices of the Institute of Child Health and Human Development. Internationally, any funding for family planning falls under the Agency for International Development.

Federal policy toward programs depends on the current political and attitudinal milieu, not only toward fertility control but also toward abortion. The competition for attention with other current health problems (such as AIDS) and other national priorities also affects the amount of funding appropriated for family planning and contraceptive research. From 1980 to 1988, the budget allotted to contraceptive research remained relatively constant at $20.5 million per year. A noticeable drop to $17.5 million occurred in 1989, whereas funding for AIDS and genetics research had a relatively large increase (U.S. Center for Population Research, February 1990, personal communication).

Where were the physicians in the history of contraception? Medical endorsement of contraception (considered an immoral or unsafe practice) was slow. The teaching of reproductive physiology in the nineteenth century was basically ignored. As late as 1890, the prevalent attitude was advocation of large families, and any participation of physicians in contraception was deemed inappropriate. Not until 1912 did the founder of American pediatrics, Abraham Jacobi, note in his presidential address to the American Medical Association (AMA) the social obligation to encourage contraception to improve public health. William A. Pusey, in his presidential address to the AMA, suggested that birth control be endorsed not only for medical reasons but also for eugenic considerations and to reduce population. Neither gained much attention. As late as 1936, a special committee of the AMA denounced lay birth-control organizations and programs. Birth control had remained largely outside the medical profession. When the AMA finally endorsed contraception in 1937, it was mainly to guard against useless and possibly injurious techniques and to maintain control over quackery (Speert 1980).

Contraceptive Techniques

Natural Methods

The most simple contraceptive technique is abstinence. Rhythm, natural family planning, or periodic abstinence is based on the premise that female fertility is confined to an identifiable period. Coitus interruptus is the withdrawal of the penis just before or at the time of ejaculation. This is not an effective practice, since active sperm deposited immediately before withdrawal can fertilize the ovum. Coitus reservatus, the withholding of ejaculation, is unreliable for the same reason. Breast-feeding suppresses ovulation but is highly variable from woman to woman and from culture to culture, probably because of varying amounts of time spent suckling an infant. The length of the anovulatory period is thus unpredictable; the return of menses may occur after the return of ovulation, making predictability of ovulation uncertain. Allowing the infant to nurse at will throughout the day and night does decrease fertility effectively in some nontechnological cultures. The introduction of artificial milk formula has undermined this physiological process.

Barrier and Spermicidal Methods

Barrier methods of contraception include the condom, the diaphragm, the contraceptive sponge, the cervical cap, and spermicidal foams, jellies, creams, suppositories, and film. These are the most straightforward and time-tested contraceptive options. Use of the barrier methods may also provide protection against sexually transmitted infections (including gonorrhea, chlamydia, and pelvic inflammatory disease) and cervical neoplasia. Readers will be familiar with the condom and diaphragm. The vaginal contraceptive sponge is a pillow-shaped polyurethane sponge containing 1 gram of nonoxynol-9 spermicide. The cervical cap is a cup-shaped device that fits over the cervix and is held partially in place by suction between its firm flexible rim and the surface of the cervix or the upper vaginal wall. Use of vaginal spermicides may also help prevent transmission of the AIDS virus because of their lethal effect on the human immunodeficiency virus (HIV) in vitro. For this reason, the spermicidal latex condom is considered an ideal protection against HIV transmission.

Intrauterine Devices

The discontinuation of production and distribution of most intrauterine devices (IUDs) was provoked by product-liability litigation, but the IUD remains a medically sound and excellent method. Among some suggestions of mechanisms of action are an inflammatory response causing lysis of the blastocyst and sperm or prevention of implantation. The IUD is believed to increase local production of prostaglandins that inhibit implantation. Copper devices compete with zinc, which inhibits carbonic anhydrase and possibly alkaline phosphatase activity. Copper may also interfere with estrogen uptake and its intracellular effects on the endometrium. Progestin-elaborating IUDs disrupt proliferative secretory maturation, causing endometrial suppression and impairing implantation (Hatcher et al. 1988).

Hormonal Methods: Precoital

Hormonal control of ovulation implantation, gamete transport, and corpus luteum function has resulted in the development of oral contraceptives (OCs). These widely used preparations consist of synthesized estrogens and progestins. Each preparation has a specific configuration of estrogenic, progestational, and androgenic activity. Reports of adverse reactions and complications associated with OCs include nausea, breast tenderness or enlargement, cyclic weight gain caused by fluid retention, leukorrhea, cervical extrophia, headaches, thromboembolic disorders, pulmonary emboli, cerebrovascular accidents, hepatocellular adenomas, hepatocellular leiomyomas, and telangiectasia. The progestin, with its androgenic and progestational effects, may result in increased appetite and weight gain, fatigue, depression, decreased libido, acne, breast enlargement, decreased carbohydrate tolerance, diabetogenesis, headaches, pruritus, increased low-density lipoprotein cholesterol levels, and decreased high-density lipoprotein cholesterol levels (Hatcher et al. 1988). It is not clear which of the components of the OCs cause which complications.

Subdermal implants are being marketed in the United States. Norplant implants are nonbiodegradable Silastic plastic rods containing levonorgestrel. A series of six hollow capsules, each the size of a 1-inch toothpick, are filled with 36 milligrams of levonorgestrel and surgically implanted in the skin of a woman's upper arm through a 2-millimeter incision. The implant can be removed when a pregnancy is desired or the dosage is depleted. Norplant users appear to have protection against infection and 96.6% effectiveness after 1 year. The main complaint from users is the disruption of menstrual cycles (Singh et al. 1988). Biodegradable implants that never have to be removed are being developed (Hatcher et al. 1988).

Monthly injectable contraceptives combining estrogen and a progestin are widely used in some countries. The hormones are suspended in a solution that is injected each month,without disruption of the menstrual cycle. Injectable microspheres and microcapsules contain tiny particles of hormone attached to polymers of different sizes, suspended in a solution and injected. For 1–6 months, a constant effective dose is delivered. This method will be available in the United States in the 1990s. A levonorgestrel-impregnated vaginal ring, releasing a 3-month supply of hormone, should also be available soon (Hatcher et al. 1988).

Postcoital Techniques

Postcoital contraceptive techniques include morning-after pills. These include the combined birth-control pills, which contain 50 micrograms of ethynyl estradiol and 9.5 milligrams of DL-norgestrel (Ovral, a product marketed in the United States), and a high-dose oral estrogen, such as diethylstilbestrol (DES). Both have a low failure rate, but Ovral has fewer adverse side effects. When Ovral is used as the morning-after pill, two tablets are taken within 72 hours (preferably within 12–24 hours) of intercourse. Two more tablets are taken 12 hours later. Bleeding usually occurs within 21–30 days. Although DES was formerly an option for postcoitus contraception, it is no longer approved in the United States for that use because of the risk of teratogenic effects and malignancy in the offspring in the event of a method failure.

Progesterone antagonists (RU-486) prevent the progesterone effect and disrupt the stability of the endometrium. RU-486 prevents implantation or causes sloughing of a fertilized zygote. When taken orally within 10 days of the expected onset of the missed menstrual period, RU-486 produces a complete abortion in 85% of women using the method (Cousinet et al. 1986).

Morning-after IUD insertion prevents ovum implantation. The device should be inserted within 5–7 days of unprotected intercourse. It is usually not suitable for nulliparous women, and women who have multiple sexual partners, who have been raped, or who have a recent history of pelvic inflammatory disease. Menstrual extraction may be performed if the expected menses is as late as 2 weeks. A positive diagnosis of pregnancy should be made, unless the patient wishes to avoid the problem of dealing with issues of abortion. The procedure has a low cost and can be done on an outpatient basis with no cervical dilatation, no anesthesia, and minimal risk when performed by a properly trained staff. The method is that of a vacuum aspiration of uterine contents through a sterile plastic cannula inserted into the endometrial cavity (Hatcher et al. 1988).

Methods Being Developed

Other methods of contraception being developed include plans for an antifertility vaccine to disrupt gestation and battery-operated intracervical implants that deter sperm migration by setting up a weak electric current across the cervix (Hatcher et al. 1988). Current male contraception research appears to be directed at inhibition of steroid and sperm production (Linde et al. 1981).

Postpregnancy Contraception

Immediate postpartum contraceptive options include lactation, sterilization, IUD insertion (not customary practice in the United States because of the risk of an increased expulsion rate and of uterine perforation and infection), and hormonal methods. Oral contraceptives may begin as early as the fifth postpartum day. Lactating mothers are advised not to use OCs while breast-feeding because of milk transmission of OCs; they should wait until their infants are weaned before initiating hormonal methods. Diaphragm fitting requires a period of waiting until vaginal relaxation is reduced to normal (Keith et al. 1979).

The considerations for initiating postabortal contraception are similar to those for initiating postpartum contraception. The involutional changes require less time, and the risks of hemorrhage, infection, subinvolution, and thrombosis are greatly reduced. The postabortal period is an ideal time to begin contraception. The patient is likely to wish to return to sexual activity, with a strong motivation to avoid another unwanted pregnancy. Statements about postpartum oral contraception also hold for initiation of the first-trimester postabortion state. For second-trimester abortions the time for return of vaginal relaxation is similar to the postpartum situation, and certain barrier methods may have to wait until the vaginal vault allows for proper fitting (Keith et al. 1979).

Sterilization

The most reliable contraception methods are sterilization of the female by tubal ligation and hysterectomy and of the male by vasectomy. No method has met Dickinson's (1950) five criteria for the ideal contraceptive: dependability, acceptability, harmlessness, simplicity, and cheapness. In the absence of a perfect method of birth control, selection of any given method must consider effectiveness, safety, and acceptability, and it must be tailored to meet the needs of individual situations.

Cultural and Psychodynamic Factors in Fertility Control

If humankind is to live beyond murder, famine, and disease by controlling population, then family planning as defined by the World Health Organization (1971)—"a way of thinking and living that is adopted voluntarily upon the basis of knowledge, attitudes and responsible decision by individuals and couples"—must prevail. The distinction between sexuality and reproductivity is still not well understood cognitively or accepted psychologically by many people in both developed and developing areas. Because confusion, myths, and value systems based on cultural and agrarian standards exist even in the face of rapidly developing technology, effective birth control still cannot be realized.

Changing Gender Roles

In some cultures, the feminine position is viewed as a breeding organism. Women are unentitled to eroticism and sexually serve the males, who are not only enhanced in their masculinity by sexual prowess but also glorified in their reproductive capacity by inseminating. Fecundity in the female is valued; eroticism (an acknowledgment of the clitoral rather than vaginal/uterine function) is not valued but scorned. A "woman of pleasure" is a woman of ill repute. To allow sexual freedom for the female (who is actually physiologically designed with a capacity for a higher frequency of sexual responsitivity) is to jeopardize the integrity of her family. The female is also the nurturer of the young, on whom the future of the economy depends.

In such cultures, sexual pleasure for the female is associated with guilt. Control of and knowledge of the female's own body is prohibited. Masturbation (self-stimulatory experiences that may give a sense of control over one's own pleasurable responses) is disallowed. Women grow up to be ashamed of their bodies and of looking at and exploring their own anatomy. They maintain a childlike innocence in public regarding sexual and reproductive matters. Modesty is the respectable norm. Women are expected to relinquish control and decision making in favor of the passive role equated with femininity.

Sex and pregnancy have more meaning than population enhancement or control. They are outlets for love, hate, guilt, and control. Unconscious conflicts give rise to the paradox that rational behavior is expected but is not realized. The agrarian cultural ideals for womanhood conflict with the realities of social change associated with the industrialized world. The struggle of women for power over their own destiny—domestic and economic—has exploded into a significant conflict with male partners, resulting in a high frequency of divorce and disruption of family cohesiveness and support for offspring. Couple issues enter into contraceptive choice.

When parties have a healthy communication, the likelihood of contraception failure is less than in situations of conflict over control, over use of a pregnancy to cement a deteriorating relationship, or over a power struggle.

Adolescent Sexuality

Children in the United States are influenced by media presentations of sexualized advertisements and materials directed at idealizing sexual activity. Children who are lonely or feeling isolated or abandoned often seek affection, attention, and care through premature sexual behavior, resulting in early unwanted pregnancies (see Chapter 13). Sexual activity can occur in defiance of adults, in struggles for control, or in competition with a maternal figure. The rise in sexual activity of American teenage girls has been steady for the last decade, with 16 years as the average age at first intercourse (Zelnik and Kantner 1980). Despite a general increase in contraceptive use, studies of teenage sexuality reveal that 25% of teenage women state they never use contraception. About two-thirds of the sexually active teenage women who never use contraception who become pregnant represent one-half of all teenage pregnancies. The subjects state that there is a decrease in the use of the pill because of "general nervousness" about its use. Withdrawal has become doubly popular as the initial choice of contraception, and nearly 50% have recently used diaphragm, rhythm, or withdrawal (De Witt 1980). Despite public-education attempts at family planning for teenagers to avoid unwanted pregnancies, teenagers continue to enter single parenthood with suboptimal knowledge of consequences and alternatives, and they frequently repeat the experiences of their mothers, who were born and raised in similar environments and situations.

Issues Affecting Particular Methods

Practices that inhibit intercourse may be selected by those who have intelligence, discipline, and the ability to tolerate frustration. For those following religious convictions that do not sanction artificial birth control, the solution is comfortable. This process also allows some women to feel a sense of control over their body, and periodic abstinence may result in a great desire and appreciation of intercourse. Avoidance of intimacy is also a consideration.

Coitus interruptus does not require advance preparation, and it is practiced by those who prefer risk taking and spontaneity and, perhaps, by the less experienced. Women report that this method is less gratifying and produces more anxiety. It is exceeded only by rhythm in its lack of effectiveness against pregnancy. The lack of an orgasmic endpoint is frustrating to women and may foster distrust and resentment toward a nongratifying partner.

Those practices requiring advance preparation also decrease spontaneity. Use of the condom is a concrete, visible method that appeals to those of an obsessive-compulsive nature, who can routinely check and recheck the integrity of the condom material for assurance of protection. It may play a dual role in protecting the female from semen and symbolically protecting her from fantasies of being soiled by the ejaculate, which she may construe as dirty. Premature ejaculators may find the decreased penile sensitivity helpful to prolong coital exposure. The condom may connote promiscuity. In the process of purchasing a condom, the buyer publicly declares a sexual intent. For some men, a condom may be a badge of masculinity to carry for display now and again. It is a clear acceptance of responsibility by the male.

For the female, use of a diaphragm is more common among the higher socioeconomic groups. The responsibility of fertility control is assumed by the female. The woman not only admits to having sexual exposure but chooses not to have reproductive consequences and actively prevents conception, touching her own reproductive and sexual anatomy in the process. She may use the diaphragm to avoid sexual exposure when her mate approaches her by not having a device in place when he is ready for intimacy. By the time she places the diaphragm, he may have lost interest.

Foams, sponges, jellies, creams, and film can have a messy connotation or be equated comfortably with other toiletries (such as perfumes) and be used without conflict. Douching is not as popular and is not condoned by the medical community, but it may be practiced by fastidious individuals who wish to wash away the "mess" or by those prone to guilt to wash away the "sin" (For 1978).

Techniques that remove responsibility from consciousness include the pill, the sponge, the IUD, implants, and injections. Devices not requiring a decision to engage in each sexual or reproductive act appeal to the more sexually inhibited, less self-confident individual who relinquishes responsibility to the physician or to external factors. The injections and implants avoid the necessity to touch or to relate to the genitalia while considering a sexual act.

Psychopathology and Contraception

The fear of pregnancy can evoke depressive responses. Recognition of the unconscious wish for pregnancy often explains the paradox in ineffective contraceptive usage. Some women experience guilt when contraception is successful. The feminine ideal of fecundity persists strongly even in the era of the liberated woman. After achieving a successful career and economic stability, some nulliparous women approaching 35 years of age become obsessively anxious to become pregnant before they lose their reproductive potential.

Use of contraceptive methods in the mentally ill will be determined by the nature of the psychopathology and the extent to which the individual can tolerate the devices or comply with the methods of control. For instance, in borderline patients or patients with schizophrenia—those with a poor sense of boundaries—the use of a foreign object such as an IUD may be intolerable. Noncompliance will undermine the use of birth-control pills or any other method requiring consistency. Sterilization raises ethical problems. People without fertility-choice behavior may contribute to a major unresolved problem—begetting children for whom appropriate parenting is not available. Recommendation of a contraceptive entails an awareness of the emotional needs of the patient and the nature of the method chosen. To arrive at the goal of overall population control and maximum quality of life entails understanding the complex psychodynamic, social, economic, and cultural factors that influence choice in childbearing.

References

Brown JL: Hunger in the U.S. Sci Am 256:37–41, 1987

Coale AJ: Recent trends in fertility in less developed countries. Science 221:828–832, 1983

Cousinet B, LeStrat N, Ulmann A, et al: Termination of early pregnancy by the progesterone antagonist RU 486 mifepristone. N Engl J Med 315:1565–1608, 1986

De Witt K: Studies find increase in teen-age sex. New York Times, October 17, 1980, p 24

Dickinson RL: Techniques of Conception Control. Baltimore, MD, Williams & Wilkins, 1950

For CV: Psychological factors influencing the choice of contraceptive method. Medical Aspects of Human Sexuality 12:98–109, 1978

Freedman R, Berelson B: The human population. Sci Am 231:3139, 1974

Hatcher RA, Guest F, Stewart F, et al: Contraceptive Technology: 1988–1989. New York, Irvington, 1988

Keith L, Labbok M, Petty J, et al: Postpartum and Postabortal Contraception. Pittsburgh, PA, Synapse, 1979

Keyfitz N: The growing human population. Sci Am 261:119–126, 1989

Linde R, Doelle GC, Alexander N, et al: Reversible inhibition of testicular steroidgenesis and spermatogenesis by a potent gonadotropin-releasing hormone agonist in normal men. N Engl J Med 305:663–667, 1981

Singh K, Viegas DA, Ratnam SS: Norplant contraceptive subdermal implants: one year experience in Singapore. Contraception 37:457–469, 1988

Speert H: Contraception, Abortion and Sterilization in Obstetrics and Gynecology: A History. Chicago, IL, American College of Obstetrics and Gynecology, 1980

Vining DR: The growth of core regions in the Third World. Sci Am 252:40–42, 1985

Westoff CF: Marriage and fertility in the developed countries. Sci Am 239:51–57, 1978

Westhoff CF, Bumpass L: The revolution in birth control practices of U.S. Roman Catholics. Science 179:41–44, 1973

World Health Organization: Health Education in Health Aspects of Family Planning (Technical Report Series 483). Geneva, World Health Organization, 1971

Zelnik M, Kantner JF: Sexual activity, contraceptive use and pregnancy among metropolitan-area teenagers, 1971–1979. Fam Plann Perspect 12:230–237, 1980

Chapter 7

Issues in Decision Making: Psychotherapeutic Work With Women Who Have Problem Pregnancies

Elisabeth K. Herz, M.D.

An unintended pregnancy or a prenatal diagnosis of fetal abnormality creates a life crisis for the individuals concerned. The legalization of abortion allows for the termination of such a pregnancy and, for many, creates the dilemma of choice. The poignancy of the dilemma will depend on various factors. The untimely conception of an eventually planned child in a stable marriage will have emotional repercussions different from those caused by an unintended pregnancy resulting from contraceptive failure for a single student. The dilemma can become agonizing when a previously infertile couple learns that their fetus has a genetic defect with unknown consequences.

Although her partner's preference will have considerable influence on a woman's decision, the choice is ultimately hers—even if she submits to coercion by significant others. Her life will be more affected by the choice she makes, even with a supportive partner. Her basic conflict is between the responsibility for a child who may overtax her resources in the current life circumstances and the responsibility she has for herself or for the care of previous children.

Emotions are often in direct conflict with reason or preconceived notions. A strong desire to have a child can concur with a stage in life that precludes responsible motherhood. Women who had fought for freedom of choice may find, to their surprise, that they are emotionally unable to apply the right to choose abortion to themselves. To relinquish a child for adoption is, for many women, also emotionally unacceptable. To give priority to their own interests may seem unacceptably selfish and, therefore, reprehensible to many women. Not to hurt others is the moral code that guides many of us through difficult decisions. Fear of regret, torturing guilt, and later punishment for failing to adhere to this moral code can weigh heavily against the realities of a woman's current life situation, which may be adverse to unplanned motherhood.

The fundamental dilemma is that none of the alternatives represents a solution without hurt or sacrifice and potentially long-lasting consequences. The more evenly balanced the weight of the pros and cons for either choice, the more difficult it becomes to decide. Time pressure, repercussions for significant others, the unpredictability of determinant factors (such as future ability to conceive), and an overwrought emotional state can render a person incapable of making a decision.

The help required in the decision-making process is to sort out the pertinent issues in an organized manner and to assist the woman or couple in making the less detrimental choice for the future. For most women and couples this role can be carried out by a specially trained counselor, but a psychiatrist should also be able to fill such a role for his or her own patients. To do so requires an interactive crisis-intervention approach. Furthermore, the expertise of a psychiatrist is required for those women who are at risk of severe psychological sequelae.

History

Kraepelin (1909) postulated that abortion alleviated rather than precipitated a psychiatric disorder. The controversy about this issue has continued ever since (Blumberg and Golbus 1975; Crowley and Laidlaw 1967; Gluckman 1971; Kummer 1963; MacDonald 1976; Pearce 1957).

The literature of the 1960s and early 1970s was no help in predicting the outcome of pregnancy termination. A profusion of publications about the psychological consequences of abortion appeared at the time of legalization. Depending on the authors' views, the methodology, and the social environment, the reported frequency of detrimental postabortion sequelae ranged from none to almost always (Rhoads et al. 1989).

After years of experience, the World Health Organization (1978) summarized international findings as follows: "There is now a substantial body of data reported from many countries after careful and objective follow-up, suggesting frequent psychological benefits and a low incidence of adverse psychological sequelae; moreover when post-abortion depression does occur, it is often apparently due to stresses other than the abortion" (p. 22). Other studies have reached the same conclusion (Bracken and Kasl 1975a, 1975b; Callahan 1970; Cates 1982; Ford et al. 1971; Forssman and Thuwe 1966; Kris and Carmichael 1957; Moseley et al. 1981; Pearce 1957; Whittington 1970). Several other long-term studies have shown that children born of unwanted pregnancies are more prone to problems than planned children, and mandatory motherhood can be harmful to a woman's psychosocial well-being (Forssman and Thuwe 1966; Hook 1963; Matejcek et al. 1978; McCance et al. 1977; Walter 1970). As long as a woman needed a medical or psychiatric indication for obtaining a legal abortion, her psychiatrist was a powerful "gatekeeper." The interpretation of *psychiatric indication* varied from suicidality to emotional distress. Furthermore, it is hard to imagine that personal bias did not play a role in such an assessment. For instance, in an article about the psychiatrist's role in therapeutic abortion, Bolter (1962) wrote, "We have no business allowing our personal feelings about the moral or social or economic position of our patients to influence our decisions concerning therapeutic abortions" (p. 314). In the same article, however, he declared, "Despite protest to the contrary, we know that woman's main role here on earth is to conceive, deliver, and raise children. Despite all other sublimated types of activities, this is still [her] primary role" (p. 315). Many psychiatrists were relieved when the U.S. Supreme Court *Roe v. Wade* (1973) decision shifted the right to decide about elective abortion.

The New Role of Psychiatrists

Research since the *Roe v. Wade* (1973) decision has focused on predictive factors for women at risk of developing a postabortion reaction more serious than brief self-limited emotional distress (Ashton 1980; Belsey et al. 1977; Jacobsson and Palm 1974). These selected high-risk women would benefit from in-depth psychosocial counseling and care by a psychiatrist.

A new function of psychiatrists is to respond to a woman's or couple's request for help in the decision-making process. In my view, professional ethics entitle a therapist to his or her own opinion but do not allow a psychiatrist to promote this opinion through persuasion, suggestion, or manipulation. If abortion is contrary to his or her values, then it is appropriate for the therapist to disqualify himself or herself from this kind of counseling. Just as important, a clinician who acts as a counselor must scrupulously avoid inserting any prejudices in favor of abortion in general or in a specific case.

Deliberately refraining from influencing a woman with one's own opinion must not be confused with value-free psychotherapy. In my opinion, the medical professional who undertakes to facilitate the decision-making process by definition must be pro-choice. He or she professes implicitly his or her belief in the value of a person's autonomy, which includes freedom in reproductive choice as it pertains to a nonviable fetus. Opponents of abortion who hold that the right to life has superior value confer equal "personhood" to the woman and the fetus from the moment of conception. Abortion becomes synonymous with killing and consequently cannot be a choice. These two value systems are mutually exclusive.

Right-to-life proponents uphold their value system when they firmly advise against abortion under all circumstances. On the other hand, proponents for freedom of choice would usurp their professed value system by recommending a course of action. For an ambivalent woman or couple seeking help, a therapist's advice is tantamount to a prescription and interferes in the autonomous decision-making process. This does not mean that blatantly unrealistic fantasies or omitted factors on the part of the counselee must not be pointed out or corrected with facts. It is the duty of a counselor—by drawing on his or her experience and knowledge—to mention potential pitfalls of the various choices as they pertain to a woman or couple. To me, it is hubristic to assume (or deceptive to pretend) that one knows the best choice for another individual.

A clinician's strong feelings for or against a contemplated abortion deserve careful scrutiny to avoid countertransference. The choice can carry a powerful emotional charge for a therapist for personal reasons. For instance, a woman therapist who recently miscarried a wanted pregnancy may feel angry and judgmental toward another woman who considers elective abortion, or a counselor may avoid pointing out detrimental aspects of whatever choice she made for fear of reviving her own regrets. It may also appeal to a clinician's narcissism to be put in the role of the adviser. It is essential to remember that a counselor represents an authority figure for a woman torn between the pros and cons of abortion. Any opinion expressed by the counselor for or against abortion has the weight of professional advice, which the woman will tend to follow. The recommendation will short-circuit her own deliberations, allow her to avoid dealing with her conflicting feelings, and hand the responsibility to the authority figure who made the decision for her. Without the painful process of working through the conflict and making her own choice, the woman is ill-prepared for the consequences. It is the woman who must live with the consequences of the decision for the rest of her life and with her own psychosocial resources, which are unquestionably different from those of her counselor. Therefore, the choice must be that of the woman or couple, and skilled assistance in the decision-making process can help to prevent subsequent psychiatric morbidity.

Risk Factors for Postdecisional Problems

Risk factors seem to predispose a woman or couple to postdecision regret. These risk factors fall into five main categories:

1. A high degree of ambivalence is correlated with statistical significance to later regret (Blumberg and Golbus 1975; Blumberg et al. 1975; Bracken and Kasl 1975a, 1975b; Friedman et al. 1974; Kapor-Stanulovic 1972; Patt et al. 1969). Delay in seeking an abortion until the second trimester is a warning signal and is frequently caused by conscious or unconscious ambivalence (Bracken and Kasl 1975a, 1975b). Undergoing the procedure so late carries a greater risk of serious psychological sequelae than if the procedure were performed during the first trimester (Friedman et al. 1974; Kaltreider 1973), but we have no evidence that the risk is greater than carrying an unintended pregnancy to term. Availability of nonjudgmental counseling may prevent the delay. Frequent repeaters are especially in need of in-depth psychiatric exploration, which may uncover conflicts beyond the abortion issue. Many women, torn by conflict in the decision-making process, are well aware of their ambivalence and reach out for help.

2. Psychosocial instability, poor support (Ford et al. 1971; Friedman et al. 1974; Niswander and Patterson 1967), and coercion by significant others (Blumberg and Golbus 1975; Ekblad 1955; Friedman et al. 1974; Patt et al. 1969; Watters 1980) also increase the risk of a negative outcome. These factors indicate a preexisting vulnerability. The additional crisis can overtax a pregnant woman's ability to adjust.

3. Improved obstetrical care makes maternal health factors a rare indication for pregnancy termination. Conception in spite of rational awareness that a pregnancy may have disastrous health consequences for her may indicate a woman's desire for a child, but it may also be an attempt to ignore her disorder. Termination becomes a painful reminder of her physical limitations and carries the risk of subsequent emotional disturbance (Blumberg and Golbus 1975; Pare and Raven 1970).

4. Prenatal diagnosis of a defective fetus creates an acute emotional crisis and can have long-lasting consequences for both partners (Blumberg and Golbus 1975). The intellectual awareness of the purpose for amniocentesis, to detect a genetic defect, does not prepare a couple for the trauma when it actually happens. Making the decision for or against abortion becomes especially agonizing when the extent of the child's handicap is unpredictable, such as in Down's syndrome. Furthermore, it is worse when a woman is close to the end of her reproductive years or has infertility problems. Even when selective abortion is rationally accepted, the emotional resolution is extremely difficult for many reasons including the fact that the child was desired, bonding is advanced by the second trimester, and there has been public awareness of the pregnancy. The newer method of chorionic villi sampling, performed at 9 weeks of gestation, has obvious advantages, but it carries a higher risk of accidental interruption of a pregnancy (Rhoads et al. 1989).

Shame about passing on inferior genetic material, fear of future problems, guilt about transgression of moral values, and other compounding personal factors can also play a role. The strain can disrupt a marital relationship, compounding the emotional distress. Comprehensive medical care after an abortion of a defective fetus certainly should include crisis intervention and supportive therapy.

5. Prior or concomitant psychiatric disorders may adversely affect the outcome of elective abortion. Women with mild psychiatric problems do not seem to differ statistically from control subjects in their emotional reactions (Ewing and Rouse 1973), but a few cases of postabortion recurrence have been reported in women with histories of previous psychoses. The establishment of a causal relationship is difficult. No one knows what the outcome of a term pregnancy would have been for a woman who had an abortion (Ford et al. 1971; Gluckman 1971; Meyerowitz et al. 1971).

The presence of severe preexisting or ongoing psychopathology can make it difficult for a psychiatrist to exercise professional restraint and refrain from interjecting his or her own opinion. Chaotic life circumstances, nonexistent support systems, lack of compliance with medication, impaired means of cognitive assessment, and other maternal psychosocial problems raise unavoidable concerns for a prospective child. Consistent contraception itself is unmanageable for some psychiatric patients, resulting in repeated abortions.

The previously held opinion that women with severe psychopathology are less fertile was found to be invalid after many previously institutionalized women had been released into the community. A psychiatrist must convey the current knowledge of risk factors of psychiatric sequelae, postabortion as well as postpartum. A patient needs to be informed that the teratogenic effect of psychotropic drugs in the first trimester is still not satisfactorily clarified and creates a potential risk for her child.

In their monumental review of 105 studies, Goldberg and DiMascio (1978) found that the evidence demonstrates "the relative safety for the fetus and newborn of psychotropic drugs administered to pregnant women" (p. 1053). Despite this conclusion, caution—especially in the first trimester—is urged; there are strong warnings about teratogenicity concerning specific drugs such as lithium and benzodiazepines. Furthermore, this review does not include the large French multicenter prospective survey by Rumeau-Rouquette et al. (1977), who found: "There was a significant excess of malformed infants when women had taken phenothiazines during the first three months after the last menstrual period" (p. 57). Furthermore, "These data are to be added to results of recent surveys showing a significant increase of malformations in children exposed in utero to anticonvulsants, carbamates, benzodiazepines, tricyclic antidepressants, and amphetamines" (p. 57). The relevant references for those studies are included in the article.

Edlund and Craig (1984) published an epidemiological reevaluation that pointed out severe methodological shortcomings common to practically all studies. The statistical reanalysis of the methodologically soundest study, by Milkovich and Van den Berg (1976), comes to a conclusion opposite that of these authors, who postulated the absence of demonstrable teratogenicity. The reanalysis found that there is an increase of fetal anomalies in women taking psychotropic medication, especially if the medication is used between 4 and 10 weeks postfertilization. This finding is particularly disquieting because it occurred in psychiatrically healthy women who took the drugs mainly for antiemetic reasons in much smaller dosages than are necessary for psychiatric therapy.

The results of studies on psychotic postpartum women also demonstrate conflicting outcomes regarding the effect of major tranquilizers on a fetus. All of the studies, however, show that children of women with severe psychopathology have a much higher rate of fetal defects, such as brain malformations and perinatal mortality, than the general population, regardless of drug intake (Edlund and Craig 1984; Kris and Carmichael 1957; Rieder et al. 1975; Simon and Senturia 1966).

If her history indicates that a patient will require drugs during the full duration of her pregnancy, she needs to be aware that psychotropic drugs taken in the third trimester or during lactation can also cause neonatal complications.

To make an informed decision about her pregnancy, a patient also needs to know that the recurrence rate of severe preexisting mental illness in the postpartum phase is high (Brockington and Kumar 1982; Inwood 1985). Such recurrence is especially frequent in bipolar and schizoaffective disorders and, to a lesser extent, in schizophrenia. The stress of adjusting to parenthood can also result in a brief psychotic break in an individual with a borderline personality disorder.

In countries like Denmark, persons with certain medical hereditary disorders can only obtain a marriage license after sterilization. The system in the United States is based on the least possible interference of government in an individual's life and respects the right of a person to reproductive choice. A psychiatrist, too, must respect this right in his or her work with a patient.

The tragic cases of psychotic women impregnated without consent and incompetent to decide for or against abortion represent a societal issue that extends beyond the purview of psychiatrists alone. A psychiatrist should act as an adviser to a standing bioethical committee that can be called on short notice. Such an interdisciplinary group would be the most useful forum to address the medical, social, legal, and ethical issues in such cases in the context of a patient's mental state. Given the current social climate, after the previous excesses of involuntary sterilization of female inmates at psychiatric institutions, an abortion without consent of a mental patient is probably difficult to attain.

The Decision-Making Process

The theoretical work on decision making under conflict by Janis (1968) and Janis and Mann (1968) is useful preparation for the professional who chooses to do this kind of intervention. They described five stages of the process: 1) acknowledging the problem; 2) awareness of options for the solution; 3) weighing pros and cons; 4) bolstering the most attractive alternative; and 5) acting on the decision.

A woman or couple seeking help has already acknowledged the unwanted or defective pregnancy and is aware of the three alternatives: carrying to term and keeping the baby, carrying to term and relinquishing the baby for adoption, and inducing abortion. The third stage of weighing pros and cons and then contrasting them to achieve (according to Janis and Mann) "maximization of net gains" and "minimization of serious losses" frequently poses the greatest problem. Advantages and disadvantages of the alternatives are examined in terms of the values they hold and the "anticipated utilitarian gains or losses for significant others and self" and "anticipated approval or disapproval of others and self" (Janis and Mann 1968, p. 335). What this really means is how the actions of the woman or couple would do violence to their values and beliefs.

A counselor's role is to assist a woman or couple by bringing additional considerations to their attention pertaining to the aforementioned vulnerability factors. Individual pertinent factors of a woman's formative years need to be made accessible to her awareness. The counselor must also emphasize long-term and short-term issues (e.g., a teenager's paralyzing fear of her parent's reaction) and must stress that avoidance can lead to a decision by default. In addition, the counselor needs to encourage the woman or couple to live out one choice in their imagination as if it were already accomplished and to ascertain how it feels. They can then rehearse the alternative choice, going back and forth until the single best alternative emerges.

In the fourth stage of this process, the woman or couple leans toward one choice and bolsters selectively the most attractive alternative. The counselor has to ensure that negative factors that could otherwise enhance postdecisional regret are not overlooked. Acting on the decision is the fifth and last stage. It can be delayed if the woman or couple ambivalently reverts to previous stages or if new factors become apparent. Prolonged delay, naturally, becomes a decision.

In summary, in the short time available, a woman or couple needs crisis intervention with a problem-solving approach based on sorting out the pertinent issues to reach a deliberate—and deliberated—decision.

Clinical Approach

I now present my method, which has been developed by trial and error in my extensive clinical work as an obstetrician, gynecologist, and psychiatrist. I find it essential to introduce a structure based on a framework of relevant questions, much as such a framework is used in making a differential diagnosis. These questions address potential risk factors for later regret. It is helpful to address the concrete reality issues before moving to the emotional implications of the different alternatives.

Here is an example for a model of the first session with a woman who comes for help.

Schema

1. What is the woman's life situation? Age? Time of gestation? Physical status? Marital status? Children? Work? No work? Finances?
2. Is the prospective father in the picture? What effect does his presence or absence have on the couple's relationship? What is the woman's anticipated guess about his reaction? Will she get support from him, relatives, or friends? For which decision? Outside pressure or coercion?
3. Were there previous losses or difficult decisions? How did the woman cope? Was there previous depression? Suicide attempts?
4. What is the woman's family background? Relationship to her mother? What values has she internalized in the formative years? What were her own life plans and goals? Which way would they be affected?

As the next step, I suggest a procedure that I adopted from decision theory. On the basis of the information gathered in this session, a list of pros and cons is prepared. I ask the woman to assign to every factor an emotional weight on a scale of 1 to 10 to help her clarify their relative importance. This list serves as the basis for our next session and can be expanded when new information or developments surface. The scheduling will depend on the time constraint; every effort must be made for the woman or couple's decision before the end of the first trimester. Any termination after this date carries considerably higher risks for the patient. Therefore, any clinician should first consider if he or she can take on this task, which involves time-intensive work.

It is useful to recommend keeping the list of pros and cons for times of subsequent doubt about choice. It serves as a reminder as to why the decision was made for choice A and not for choice B. Factors arguing against choice B are easily forgotten, and the pros for choice B become magnified while one struggles with the cons of the choice taken. There is no ideal solution for a highly conflicted choice, and adjusting comfortably to the consequences can sometimes be difficult, if not impossible.

Case Example

A.R. is a 35-year-old married woman. She is in the ninth week of her first pregnancy, which occurred through contraceptive failure. Several years ago she was told that she had endometriosis and that this diminished her chances of conception. She married 6 months ago. She and her husband recently lost important positions because of a takeover of their firm. Thus there are financial problems.

A.R. describes herself as a "career-oriented feminist" and "not very interested in having a child." Her self-identity is linked to the high achievements in her career, and especially now, when she has to be able to make a new start, she needs to be in command of all of her faculties. Who is going to employ a pregnant woman in a powerful position?

Since A.R. is married and has a close and warm relationship with her husband, both want to have a child eventually. Given the circumstances, her husband is also ambivalent now.

She feels frightened, shocked, trapped, and hostile toward this pregnancy. To her, a child means sacrifice of personal freedom, career opportunities, a life-style that she describes as "self-indulgent and Bohemian," and time with her husband. The pregnancy is, therefore, an interference—a threat—to her.

Although she is rationally in favor of a woman's right to abortion, to her the step seems like "killing." She tends to be prone to guilt and had been in therapy for a depression. She is afraid of a recurrence.

She is the only child of a workaholic father and a mother who had to give up her own profession when she became pregnant. The parents had a poor marital relationship, and A.R. felt very early that her father preferred her company to that of her mother. She is afraid that her husband might also prefer the child, and she already sees it as a rival for his affection.

Her age and the endometriosis speak for continuation of the pregnancy, and she does wish to have her husband's child. A.R. feels so torn that she is unable to make a decision. I suggested a joint session with her husband, who was described as totally opposed to psychiatry but came anyway.

B.E. is a 32-year-old man who related that he went from total rejection of this pregnancy to "good feelings" about it, swinging wildly between extremes, and felt numb and unable to come to any decision. He thinks that the decision should be made jointly, but he also thinks that more weight should be given to his wife's preference.

A child means for him an important life experience that he would not like to miss. He had always had good relationships with children, and he likes to stay in touch with youth.

Financial concerns worry him, but they are probably not insurmountable.

He grew up as the second of three boys in an emotionally distant family. He believes he could be a better parent than his own; it would be a challenge to prove that to himself.

In his opinion, his wife would make a "terrific" mother, but they would have to make "space" in their lives for the child, and although he means to participate in the child care, his wife would have the greater burden.

On the basis of our sessions, we prepared a list of pros and cons. I asked that for the next session each of them separately assign to each factor an emotional weight on a scale from 1 to 10, with the higher numbers assigned to factors with greater weight. When we compared the lists, they were surprised at how differently they weighed their concerns:

Arguments for carrying the pregnancy to term

	Wife	Husband
Age	2	3
"Killing"	7	1
Mother's example	4	2
Prospect of remaining childless	5	6
To have child of the partner	3	5
Staying in touch with youth	2	10
Fear of procedure	6	2

Arguments against carrying the pregnancy to term

	Wife	Husband
Job crisis, finances	10	8
Career impediment	6	2
Interference with their relationship	10b	7b
Loss of freedom	3	2
Uncertainty about future	5	4
Fear of "rotten kid"	2	6
Duress, lack of control	5	1

The exercise set off a dynamic process. B.E. became aware that he was more in favor of proceeding with the pregnancy than he had realized. His realization, in turn, had a decisive effect on A.R.'s preference. This device of weighing each factor had improved communication and helped to clarify the issue and move them to a mutual decision. They chose to continue the pregnancy. The wife and I worked awhile in individual therapy on unresolved conflicts with her mother and to strengthen her separation and individuation process. An annual photograph is signed as the "right choice."

Conclusion

A decision arrived at by default carries a greater risk for subsequent regret and adverse psychological consequences. When a woman or couple realizes and accepts that there is no magical solution to the conflict that an unintended or defective pregnancy may cause, then the painful and laborious process of making the least-detrimental individual decision can begin. A psychiatrist can facilitate the working through of the various emotionally charged issues and help the most conducive choice to emerge.

References

Ashton JR: The psychosocial outcome of induced abortion. Br J Obstet Gynaecol 87:1115–1122, 1980

Belsey EM, Greer HS, Lal S, et al: Predictive factors in emotional response to abortion: King's termination study—IV. Soc Sci Med 11:71–82, 1977

Blumberg BD, Golbus MS, Hanson KH: The psychological sequelae of abortion performed for a genetic indication. Am J Obstet Gynecol 122:799–808, 1975

Blumberg BD, Golbus MS: Psychological sequelae of selective abortion. West J Med 123:188–193, 1975

Bolter S: The psychiatrist's role in therapeutic abortion: the unwitting accomplice. Am J Psychiatry 19:312–316, 1962

Bracken MB, Kasl SV: Delay in seeking induced abortion: a review and theoretical analysis. Am J Obstet Gynecol 121:1008–1019, 1975a

Bracken MB, Kasl SV: Denial of pregnancy, conflict, and delayed decisions to abort, in Proceedings of the Fourth International Congress of Psychosomatic Obstetrics and Gynecology. Basel, Switzerland, Karger, 1975b

Brockington IF, Kumar R (ed): Motherhood and Mental Illness. New York, Grune & Stratton, 1982

Callahan D: Abortion: Law, Choice and Morality. London, Macmillan, 1970

Cates W: Abortion myths and realities: who is misleading whom? Am J Obstet Gynecol 142:954–956, 1982

Crowley R, Laidlaw R: Psychiatric opinion regarding abortion—preliminary report of a survey. Am J Psychiatry 124:559–562, 1967

Edlund MJ, Craig TJ: Antipsychotic drug use and birth defects: an epidemiologic reassessment. Compr Psychiatry 25:32–37, 1984

Ekblad M: Induced abortion on psychiatric grounds—a followup study of 479 women. Acta Psychiatr Scand Suppl 99:1–238, 1955

Ewing JA, Rouse BA: Therapeutic abortion and a prior psychiatric history. Am J Psychiatry 130:37–40, 1973

Ford CV, Castelnuovo-Tedesco P, Lone K: Abortion: is it a therapeutic procedure in psychiatry? JAMA 218:1173–1178, 1971

Forssman H, Thuwe I: One hundred and twenty children born after application for therapeutic abortion refused. Acta Psychiatr Scand 42:71–78, 1966

Friedman CM, Greenspan R, Mittleman F: The decision-making process and the outcome of therapeutic abortion. Am J Psychiatry 131:1332–1337, 1974

Gluckman L: Some unanticipated complications of therapeutic abortion. NZ Med J 74:71–78, 1971

Goldberg HL, DiMascio A: Psychotropic drugs in pregnancy, in Psychopharmacology: A Generation of Progress. Edited by Lipton MA, DiMascio A, Killam RF. New York, Raven, 1978, pp 1047–1055

Hook K: Refused abortion: a follow-up study of 249 women. Acta Psychiatr Scand Suppl 168:7–151, 1963

Inwood DG (ed): Recent Advances in Postpartum Psychiatric Disorders. Washington, DC, American Psychiatric Press, 1985

Jacobsson L, Palm A: Psychological femininity and legal abortion. Acta Psychiatr Scand Suppl 255:291–298, 1974

Janis IL: Stages in the decision-making process, in Theories of Cognitive Consistency: A Sourcebook. Edited by Abelson RP, Aronson E, McGuire WJ. Chicago, IL, Rand McNally, 1968, pp 577–588

Janis IL, Mann LA: A conflict theory approach to attitude change and decision making, in Psychological Foundations of Attitudes. Edited by Greenwald A. New York, Academic, 1968, pp 327–388

Kaltreider N: Psychological factors in mid-trimester abortion. Psychiatr Med 4:129–134, 1973

Kapor-Stanulovic N: Three phases of the abortion process and its influence on women's mental health. Am J Public Health 62:906–908, 1972

Kraepelin E: Psychiatrie. Leipzig, Germany, J. Barth, 1909

Kris EB, Carmichael DM: Chlorpromazine maintenance therapy during pregnancy and confinement. Psychiatr Q 31:685–690, 1957

Kummer J: Post-abortion psychiatric illness—a myth? Am J Psychiatry 119:980–983, 1963

MacDonald R: Complications of abortion. Nurs Times 63:306–307, 1976

Margolis A, Davison L, Hanson K, et al: Therapeutic abortion follow-up study. Am J Obstet Gynecol 110:243–249, 1971

Matejcek Z, Dytrych Z, Schuller V: Children from unwanted pregnancies. Acta Psychiatr Scand 57:67–90, 1978

Meyerowitz S, Satloff A, Romano J: Induced abortion for psychiatric indication. Am J Psychiatry 127:1153–1160, 1971

Milkovich L, Van den Berg BJ: An evaluation of the teratogenicity of certain anti-nauseant drugs. Am J Obstet Gynecol 125:244–248, 1976

Moseley DT, Follingstad DR, Harley H, et al: Psychological factors that predict reaction to abortion. J Clin Psychol 37:276–279, 1981

Niswander K, Patterson R: Psychologic reaction to therapeutic abortion, I: subjective patient response. Obstet Gynecol 29:702–706, 1967

Pare C, Raven H: Follow-up of patients referred for termination of pregnancy. Lancet 1:635–638, 1970

Patt S, Rappaport R, Barglow P: Follow-up of the therapeutic abortion. Arch Gen Psychiatry 20:408–414, 1969

Pearce J: Discussion: the psychiatric indication for the termination of pregnancy. Proc R Soc Med 50:321, 1957

Rhoads GG, Jackson LG, Schlesselman SE, et al: The safety and efficacy of chorionic villus sampling for early prenatal diagnosis of cytogenetic abnormalities. N Engl J Med 320:609–617, 1989

Rieder RD, Rosenthal D, Wender P, et al: The offspring of schizophrenics—fetal and neonatal deaths. Arch Gen Psychiatry 32:200–211, 1975

Roe v. Wade, 410 U.S. 113 (1973)

Rumeau-Rouquette C, Goujard J, Huel G: Possible teratogenic effect of phenothiazines in human beings. Teratology 15:57–64, 1977

Simon NM, Senturia AG: Psychiatric sequelae of abortion. Arch Gen Psychiatry 15:378–389, 1966

Walter GS: Psychological and emotional consequences of elective abortion. Obstet Gynecol 36:482, 1970

Watters WW: Mental health consequences of abortion and refused abortion. Can J Psychiatry 25:68–73, 1980

Whittington H: Evaluation of therapeutic abortion as an element of preventive psychiatry. Am J Psychiatry 126:1224–1229, 1970

World Health Organization: Induced abortion (Technical Report Series No 623). Geneva, World Health Organization, 1978

Chapter 8

Psychotherapeutic Issues Related to Abortion

Sarah L. Minden, M.D.
Malkah T. Notman, M.D.

When considering the issue of psychotherapy for abortion-related problems, the first question that arises is whether there is a distinctive postabortion syndrome that suggests a particular psychotherapeutic approach. There does not, in fact, appear to be a specific disorder, but there is a range of responses that reflect each woman's reactions to her pregnancy, the quality of her relationship with her sexual partner, her circumstances at the time of becoming pregnant, and her unique personality and life history. (The literature is reviewed in detail in Chapter 2.)

During the 1940s and 1950s, it was often argued that women who had abortions were left with lifelong feelings of guilt, shame, and depression. More systematic research during the 1960s and 1970s, however, indicated that very few women experienced adverse psychological effects (Ewing and Rouse 1973; Ford et al. 1971a, 1971b; Greenglass 1976; Illsley and Hall 1976; Jacobs et al. 1974; Marder 1970; Margolis et al. 1971; Patt et al. 1969; Payne et al. 1976; Shusterman 1979; Simon et al. 1967). (For a review emphasizing negative sequelae of abortion, see Ney and Wickett 1989.) These studies also provide support for the view expressed by Payne et al. (1976) that an unwanted pregnancy, the decision about how to handle it, and the subsequent abortion constitute a life crisis analogous to other important life events and that there is a process of psychological adjustment to the crisis that is similar to the response to other life stresses. Payne et al. (1976) wrote, "The occurrence of a stressful life event [causes] turmoil and disorganization, which in turn demand mobilization of new adaptive patterns,

119

followed by resolution and reintegration. As with other life crises, the pregnancy-abortion experience holds the potential for both progressive and regressive effects. Resolution of the dilemma of an unwanted pregnancy by means of an abortion is a dynamic process, proceeding by stages over time" (p. 725).

From a clinical perspective, then, it is important not to pathologize a woman's response to unwanted pregnancy and abortion. The adaptive process model suggests that it is normal to feel vulnerable and dependent while pregnant, to experience conflict when deciding whether to continue a pregnancy, and to feel anxious and preoccupied while trying to make this decision. It is also important for clinicians to remember that American society, even after abortion was decriminalized, has at best frowned on abortion and at worst harassed and tormented women who have had abortions. In such a social climate, it is not surprising that many women might feel that their personal decision to have an abortion conflicted with societal values or that they might experience some degree of anxiety and self-doubt. Friedman et al. (1974) pointed out that in countries where abortion was less controversial than in the United States, the literature on abortion showed fewer adverse psychiatric reactions. Indeed, where social pressure supported abortion—for example, in China, after the policy of a one-child family was instituted, or in Eastern European countries, where other contraception was unavailable—women expressed antigovernment feelings by condemning abortion.

Although there appears to be a general process of adaptation to pregnancy and abortion, the particular features of each woman's adjustment are unique. The model of grief and mourning, for example, may accurately reflect the experience of a woman who wanted a child yet chose to terminate the pregnancy after having contracted rubella, but it may not reflect the feelings of relief felt by a woman who terminated an unwanted pregnancy.

The meaning ascribed to a pregnancy and to an abortion, and the response to these events, will be determined by the individual woman's current life situation, past life experiences, coping skills, vulnerability to psychiatric illness, and personality. Several issues will be interwoven, including deep-seated attitudes regarding sexuality, pregnancy, and child rearing; the nature of her relationship with her partner; whether the abortion was freely chosen; the reason for the abortion (medical or psychosocial); the way in which the abortion was obtained; the availability of a support system; and economic factors. For example, when a pregnancy is unwanted, relief after an abortion is understandable, but when a pregnancy is desired, giving it up because of external pressure, medical necessity, or incompatible life circumstances will be associated with a sense of loss, disappointment, and anger. Even when the pregnancy is not consciously wanted there may be regret, since most women have mixed feelings and some may have unconscious wishes to carry the pregnancy to term.

The particular point in the adjustment process at which a woman seeks psychiatric treatment is also important for understanding her concerns and developing a therapeutic approach. One woman may experience conflict after learning she is pregnant and require help with making the decision to carry or terminate the pregnancy. Another may be troubled by painful feelings soon after an abortion, whereas a third may feel distress many years after the event. Some women present with specific concerns about an abortion; for others, these concerns may emerge only during the course of psychotherapy initiated for other reasons (Kent et al. 1978; Ney and Wickett 1989).

The concept of a dynamic process of adjustment, then, shaped by an individual woman's psychological makeup, provides a guide to clinical assessment and treatment planning. To understand why a woman comes for help when she does and what the particular issues are, a clinician must learn the specific meaning that these events hold for her and the context in which they occurred. In this chapter we present a model for understanding the process of adaptation to pregnancy and abortion that captures the experience of many women. We also discuss various clinical issues that focus on individual reactions and therapeutic approaches.

The Process of Adaptation

The process of adaptation to pregnancy and abortion can be roughly divided into five phases: pregnancy and the decision to undergo abortion; immediate reactions (until 1 month after the abortion); short-term reactions (1–6 months after the abortion); intermediate reactions (7 months to 1 year after the abortion); and long-term reactions (more than 1 year after the abortion). Research on several hundred women during these time periods in various studies suggests that at no time are adverse psychiatric reactions frequent and that in most cases, when they occur, they are either mild and time-limited or cannot be confidently attributed to the abortion itself. Despite the methodological limitations of these studies taken individually, the consistency of their findings permits us to trust their results as a group.

Pregnancy and the Decision to Terminate

If we are to understand a woman's response to abortion, we must also understand what it means to her to be pregnant, both in general and at that particular time in her life. Women's responses to pregnancy are highly varied and reflect personality and early life experiences. For some women, pregnancy is a highly desirable state, containing many gratifications: the promise of a child to nurture, a positive identification with mother, a heightened sense of womanliness, an enhancement of a relationship, and the creation of her own family. For other women, or for the same woman at another time, pregnancy may be viewed with distaste and alarm. It may be experienced as an invasion of the body or may arouse conflicting feelings about a devalued or hated mother. Some women feel too young and immature to care for a child or have plans for their lives (at that time) that make a child seem to be a burden (Osofsky et al. 1971; Shusterman 1979).

The particular circumstances whereby a woman has become pregnant will also shape her response to the pregnancy. A woman who consciously intended to become pregnant and is pleased with the pregnancy may find herself facing a decision about abortion when she learns that she has taken a medication or been exposed to an infectious disease that may produce significant birth defects. Similarly, changes in life circumstances, such as the loss of her partner through death or divorce or the development of a serious illness in herself, may cause a woman to consider terminating her pregnancy. Although the decision to terminate a pregnancy may be easier if a genetic defect such as Down's syndrome has been discovered or if life circumstances are unequivocally inimical (as they would be for a teenager), the loss of a desired pregnancy is inevitably painful and disturbing. The reasons for terminating a pregnancy may be sound, but unconscious feelings of guilt may be awakened and lead to subsequent depression. Other people, perhaps a physician, a partner, or parents, may be blamed for the circumstances that make abortion advisable and produce responses of anger and outrage.

> Anna T. was a student in Europe in the 1930s. She lived with Michael, had no particular plans to marry, and used a diaphragm somewhat haphazardly for birth control. World War II broke out, and she left Michael to work in another part of the country. She found out that she was pregnant but, feeling that she could not raise a child alone in a wartime situation, had an abortion. Eventually Anna married, but she never had children. Many years later, reviewing her life experiences in psychotherapy, she recalled the abortion with some sadness and wished that her life had been different. When her husband died, she became depressed and then focused on the abortion, wondering whether she could have raised the child in spite of her circumstances. She felt that she would have been less lonely now had she had the child. Vivid memories reminded her of how difficult it would have been during those turbulent times, and she felt more at peace with her earlier decision.

How a woman (or her partner) deals with the decision to keep or terminate a pregnancy involves several factors, including her capacity to tolerate painful affects and ambivalence; the support she receives during the decision-making phase, through the abortion, and in the immediate postabortion period; and other aspects of her own past and current life experiences.

> Mr. and Mrs. Edwards were referred for psychotherapy by a hospital's abortion counseling service because they were having great difficulty deciding whether to have an abortion. They had a 16-year-old daughter but had been unable to

conceive again after her birth and eventually were reconciled to having only one child. The couple was shocked when Mrs. Edwards became pregnant, probably as the result of effective treatment of Mr. Edwards's chronic prostatitis. Mr. Edwards, one of two children, thought of the pregnancy as a gift from the gods. Mrs. Edwards, a perfectionist and well-organized woman who was an only child, was intensely ambivalent about the pregnancy: She oscillated between feeling that she did not want her carefully ordered world disrupted and feeling confident that she could cope with another child.

The crisis was intense, with many changes of heart on both of their parts. Mrs. Edwards scheduled an abortion but then fled the hospital just before the procedure. She later returned and had the abortion, but immediately afterward both she and her husband became depressed.

During the weeks of turmoil leading to the abortion, the couple was able to talk with their therapist only about the here-and-now question of whether to have the abortion. Afterward, exploratory psychotherapy became possible. Mrs. Edwards was able to discuss her unresolved feelings about not having another child and her wishes to maintain this pregnancy. Mr. Edwards recalled that his father, a salesman, had hesitated about taking a particular train home; he took another that crashed, and he was killed. Mr. Edwards recognized that his anger at his wife's ambivalence and his deep sense of loss were related to his father's death. After some months of therapy, the couple decided that for the time being they would not try to have another child.

A woman may find herself pregnant when she neither expects nor wants to be pregnant. If a usually effective means of birth control failed or if she had been raped, for example, a woman may experience little emotional conflict in choosing to terminate a pregnancy that she did not choose in the first place. By contrast, a woman who acted out an unconscious wish to be pregnant—perhaps a teenager having difficulty separating from her mother, an unmarried woman trying to cement an uncertain relationship, or a married woman trying to resolve career conflicts—will be forced to deal consciously with issues she had sought to avoid. Pregnancy not infrequently occurs as an unconscious response to loss or stress. Patt et al. (1969), for example, found that 30 of 35 women who had abortions had not consciously planned their pregnancies and that 15 of these unplanned pregnancies occurred after a stressful event, such as a therapist's vacation, a discharge from a psychiatric hospital, divorce, the death of a parent, or increased responsibilities. Pregnancy may also result from unconscious competitive feelings or a need to feel young and attractive.

Helen R., the mother of four children, was preparing for her oldest daughter's wedding. She was 44, and her daughter was 22. She liked her future son-in-law and admired his family, although she voiced mixed feelings about their high social status. She thought that her daughter's life was going to be easier than hers had been as a new bride. She recognized a pang of envy mixed with appreciation of her daughter's vibrant young beauty.

As Mrs. R. walked down the aisle during the wedding ceremony, she felt a surge of nausea announcing her fifth pregnancy. She had been rather hazy about her use of her diaphragm in the preceding weeks. At first she attributed this to confusion from the arrangements for the wedding, but in her psychotherapy she recognized the competitive feelings that had led to an unconscious desire to have another baby—a wish to show she was still young enough to conceive and that she was more capable than the young bride, since this would be her fifth pregnancy. She also understood that another child would not resolve her competitive feelings or other mid-life issues and decided to have an abortion.

It is important to remember that even when there is little conflict involved in having an abortion, most women feel some apprehension before the actual event (Ashton 1980; Osofsky et al. 1971; Shusterman 1979). For many women, abortion involves an unfamiliar gynecological procedure with some degree of risk, pain, and disruption of daily life. Special circumstances may heighten the anxiety for a particular woman: efforts to keep the abortion secret, a second-trimester abortion, financial difficulties, or the disapproval of significant others.

Immediate Postabortion Reactions (Until 1 Month)

Many women who seek abortion do so because they simply do not want ever to have a child. Others may be more positive about having a child but believe that at this particular time in their lives it would not be good for them or the child to continue the pregnancy. Such women usually experience little or no conflict about the decision to undergo abortion and feel relieved when the pregnancy is terminated (Friedman et al. 1974; Jacobs et al. 1974; Kretzschmar and Norris 1967; Lask 1975; Niswander and Patterson 1967; Patt et al. 1969; Payne et al. 1976; Shusterman 1979; Simon et al. 1967). Ford et al. (1971a), for example, found that women with children described as "tired mothers" who underwent sterilization after terminating a pregnancy experienced a new sense of freedom in their lives after the abortion.

Certainly some women experience negative emotional reactions, such as sadness, regret, or guilt, immediately after an abortion, but research suggests that for most women these feelings resolve fairly quickly (Brody et al. 1971; Friedman et al. 1974; Jacobs et al. 1974; Kretzschmar and Norris 1967; Niswander and Patterson 1967; Osofsky et al. 1971; Payne et al. 1976; Simon et al. 1967).

According to Friedman et al. (1974), depression after abortion is related to ongoing conflict about the decision. They noted that women who were depressed 2 weeks after an abortion "actually had deep, unconscious ambivalence about their decision. They often wanted the child but felt that their life situation made this impossible. After the abortion, the continued ambivalence was expressed in fantasies about the fetus, particularly regarding its sex. Many of these women were aware of the due date. They seemed to have a stronger tendency [than other women] to imagine a place in their lives for a baby. . . . [It] does seem that a strong desire to have a baby, which may be concurrent with a woman's certainty that she is not prepared for a child at the time, contributes to this reaction. These women appear to cathect the fetus and mourn its loss. Our experience suggests that women with less negative postabortion response have cathected the fetus less" (Friedman et al. 1974, p. 1333).

Follow-up interviews conducted in the Payne et al. study (1976), however, revealed a different pattern: Very few of the women spontaneously recalled their due date, but many more remembered the anniversary of the abortion (see also Cavenar et al. 1978). Grief reactions are not uncommon among women who want to continue a pregnancy but choose to terminate it for medical reasons, such as exposure to rubella (Friedman et al. 1974; Niswander and Patterson 1967). Similarly, a woman who feels compelled to have an abortion because her husband or lover is unable or unwilling to have the baby or because her parents insist that she terminate the pregnancy may feel angry and depressed. As with other grief reactions or responses to other kinds of life stresses, feelings of sadness, emptiness and loss, tearfulness, sleeplessness, and loss of interest typically abate over the next 6–12 months. Resolution may be hastened by becoming pregnant again (Simon et al. 1967).

> Susan L., a 25-year-old single woman, sought psychiatric consultation because of panic attacks that had become more frequent and intense over the past 4 months. During the consultation she did not mention that her first attack occurred while she was being wheeled to an operating room to have an abortion. It was not until the next session that she spoke of the abortion, saying that she had decided to have it because she and her boyfriend were not ready to marry and that she had little interest in being a mother. She stated that she had felt relief immediately after the abortion and had experienced no sadness or regret. She reported that she had a second panic attack 2 weeks later when she was flying home to visit her parents.
>
> In her psychotherapy sessions during the next 6 months, Ms. L. became aware of a wish to have a child someday and a sense of loss at having terminated her pregnancy. More prominent, however, was anger at her boyfriend for his unwillingness to marry her and raise their child with her. She also recognized how frightened she was of expressing her angry feelings. She associated this fear with long-standing suppression of anger toward her parents, particularly concerning their efforts to control her decisions. There was a striking end to her panic attacks when she allowed herself to be consciously aware of her boyfriend's infidelity, confront him, and end their relationship.

Short-Term Reactions (1–6 Months)

Payne et al. (1976) demonstrated that even high levels of anxiety, depression, anger, guilt, and shame typically decline to normal or near-normal levels by the sixth month after an abortion (see also Ashton 1980; Brody et al. 1971). There is also evidence to suggest that like other major life events, pregnancy and abortion contain the potential for maturation and personal growth. The very process of making a difficult life decision like that about abortion can have positive effects on a woman's self-esteem and sense of autonomy (Ashton 1980; Gilligan 1982; Margolis et al. 1971; Payne et al. 1976). Margolis et al. (1971) interviewed 43 patients between 4 and 6 months after an abortion and found that 51% reported greater empathy and felt freer and more feminine. Many women who became pregnant because of haphazard and inadequate contraception indicated that they had developed more effective birth-control practices (see also Jacobs et al. 1974).

Of course, significant psychiatric distress can and does occur. Some women are upset at the loss of control or indication of the power of irrational impulses that an unplanned pregnancy may represent. They may become intensely self-reproachful after a contraceptive failure or other apparent mistake.

> Barbara C. had become pregnant in a casual relationship after breaking up with her boyfriend. She realized how much becoming pregnant was a reaction to losing him. Although her fantasies of having a baby comforted her and made her feel less alone, she felt that she was not able to raise a child and decided to have an abortion. She felt guilty for having become pregnant and castigated herself for being so "stupid" as not to have used contraceptives. While she was in the hospital, she felt that the nurse was critical of her and had singled her out for disapproving looks. Psychotherapy helped clarify her own conflict about the pregnancy and abortion; it enabled her to recognize that her own guilty feelings were being projected and that the guilt was related to her regret at having ended the first relationship.

Intermediate (7–12 Months) and Long-Term (More Than 12 Months) Reactions

Even patients who have symptoms of distress in the early weeks and months after an abortion generally are emotionally well by 1 year (Ashton 1980; Brody et al. 1971). There is no substantial research evidence of significant long-term negative psychological effects of abortion (Jansson 1965; Kretzschmar and Norris 1967; Pasnau 1972; Patt et al. 1969; Simon et al. 1967; Whittington 1970). Indeed, reports on women who sought psychiatric help (Greenglass 1976; Whittington 1970), required psychiatric hospitalization (Greenglass 1976; Simon et al. 1967), completed suicide (Jansson 1965), or suffered severe or chronic psychiatric symptoms (Patt et al. 1969) suggest that these women had preexisting psychiatric illnesses or adverse life experiences concurrent with the abortion that led to their difficulties and that the abortions per se were not the primary cause of their problems. Greenglass (1976) emphasized the importance of not assuming that there is a causal relationship when psychiatric difficulties occur after an abortion: Four women who attempted suicide after an abortion did so not because of the abortion, but because of problems in the relationship with the sexual partner. This, of course, does not mean that an abortion may not be a precipitating event for psychiatric decompensation in a vulnerable woman.

> Betty M. came from a religious family, but she stopped attending church when she went away to college and became caught up in the excitement of new relationships and new ideas. During her sophomore year she began to feel distant from her friends, questioned the meaning of her courses, felt her roommates were critical of her, and became interested in a religious group that offered a new orientation to nature, a healthful vegetarian diet, and an Eastern philosophy. She felt comfortable in the company of the all-encompassing group activities. She became sexually involved with one of the young men in the group, but, as part of the "natural" approach, they did not use contraceptives. When Ms. M. became pregnant, she was shocked and conflicted; neither she nor her lover felt able to raise a child. She decided to have an abortion, but afterward she felt guilty and confused. Having contravened the natural orientation of the group and the religious principles of her family by having an abortion, she felt intense guilt. She became preoccupied with the pregnancy and abortion, was unable to sleep, withdrew from her lover and the group, and dropped out of school. An old friend suggested she seek help at a nearby psychiatry clinic.
>
> During psychotherapy it became clear that Ms. M. had been ambivalent about moving away from her family. The new religious group had represented an alternative family, and she had played the role of a child in that family, in part, by becoming pregnant. In therapy she was confronted by her feelings of loss for her original family.

Whether guilt is a prominent feature in postabortion reactions has been addressed by many investigators, and there is little or no evidence that guilt or other psychiatric symptomatology arising from guilt is common.

Recognition and Assessment of Psychiatric Difficulties

Although the numbers of women with adverse reactions to abortion are few, some women have psychiatric symptoms that arise from an abortion. Several studies have indicated that relatively few women seek psychotherapy for reasons directly related to the abortion—roughly 2–14% (Ashton 1980; Barnes et al. 1971; Ewing and Rouse 1973; Kretzschmar and Norris 1967; Margolis et al. 1971), with one study reporting a high of 26% (Whittington 1970). If a woman has emotional difficulties, they may become apparent to an obstetrical clinician before, during, or immediately after the abortion or at a follow-up interview, and he or she should initiate discussion of the patient's need for help. Since the U.S. Supreme Court *Roe v. Wade* (1973) decision eliminated mandatory psychiatric evaluation before abortion, obstetrical clinicians should be familiar with the indications for mental health consultation. They should also provide routine follow-up appointments to ensure that postabortion difficulties are recognized if they occur.

Obstetrics and gynecology training programs should provide education about the psychological issues surrounding pregnancy and abortion and instruction in detecting significant psychopathology and making referrals. Most facilities performing abortions offer counseling services, and the social workers and psychiatrists associated with these services may provide ongoing education to their colleagues. Since a woman may experience psychiatric symptoms but not attribute them to an abortion directly, or may hesitate to make an abortion known, nonobstetrical physicians, nurses, and mental health professionals should include questions about pregnancies and abortions when taking medical and psychiatric histories. Ashton (1980) found that 28 of 64 women complained of emotional distress after their abortions and 23 consulted their family physician; only 11 specifically mentioned their emotional difficulties.

During the phase of deciding whether to continue a pregnancy, unusual difficulty in making a decision, intense ambivalence, family conflict, and evidence of pressure on the woman to make a particular choice all would suggest the need for mental health consultation. Obstetrical clinicians should ask each woman explicitly about her reasons for seeking an abortion, her feelings about having the abortion, and the feelings of those close to her, particularly the feelings of her sexual partner and family. The clinician should determine whether the woman is making her decision freely or is passively complying with the wishes of others. The quality of the woman's support system should be evaluated; if she lacks emotional support (perhaps because she is keeping her pregnancy secret or the conflict with her family or partner is too intense), referral to a mental health clinician is indicated. Many people would agree that young teenagers should talk with a mental health professional. (The legal and therapeutic issues specific to teenagers are addressed in Chapter 13.)

A woman with mental retardation or a major mental disorder that interferes with her ability to understand the implications of pregnancy and abortion should be referred to a psychiatrist for evaluation of her capacity to make a rational decision and to consent to the procedure. When a woman is unable to understand the implications of her decision, it will be necessary to obtain a court-appointed guardian to act on her behalf. In most cases these kinds of difficulties will be obvious, but during the initial evaluation the clinician should be attentive to abnormalities of mental status.

Indications for mental health consultation before or after an abortion include significant depression, anxiety, behavioral problems, suicidal ideation, mental retardation, and psychosis. Since some degree of depression and anxiety is common before and soon after an abortion, referral should be made for unusually severe symptoms that interfere with daily functions, sleep, or appetite; involve suicidal ideas; or persist after the immediate postabortion period. Since intense regret and guilt and painful ruminations are uncommon after abortions, these are also indications for referral.

An obstetrical clinician or associated staff should also assess each woman's contraceptive knowledge and practices and risk of future pregnancy. This should be done during the initial evaluation in the event that the woman does not return for a follow-up visit. The clinician should help the woman identify, in a nonjudgmental fashion, possible reasons for having become pregnant. If contraceptive problems exist, solutions should be offered. Some women, even if sexually active or apparently sophisticated, are uninformed or confused about conception and contraception. Others may have had a specific reason for not preventing a pregnancy, such as feeling unable to ask a partner to use a condom. Still others may have a long history of impulsive or risk-taking sexual behavior.

Too little attention is generally paid to the potential father. Although the role of the father raises many legal and moral issues, it is important for obstetrical and mental health clinicians to know the father's wishes and how the couple is handling the pregnancy, the decision about termination, and the subsequent abortion. In some instances, couple therapy is indicated or the father may be offered a referral for himself. (This issue is covered in Chapter 10.)

Predicting Women at Risk for Postabortion Psychiatric Difficulties

Although it is difficult to predict which women will have postabortion problems, research suggests some risk factors that should alert a clinician to potential problems. These predictors should not be construed as contraindications to abortion or as indications for routine preabortion counseling (Group for the Advancement of Psychiatry 1969; Pasnau 1972; Payne et al. 1976). Rather, they highlight women at risk who should be followed closely for adverse reactions and referred for psychiatric consultation if and when difficulties arise (American Psychiatric Association 1970). Where there are several risk factors present, referral before problems emerge might prevent future difficulties. It is important to remember that these risk factors are suggested by studies that may have important methodological shortcomings: small selected samples, inadequate control groups, retrospective data collection, and insufficient follow-up. Studies of demographic factors, in particular, are probably outdated; it is important to determine whether their results still hold under contemporary social conditions.

Medical Indication for Abortion

When a desired pregnancy is terminated for probable fetal abnormalities or to protect the health of the mother, many women will experience a grief reaction, according to Niswander and Patterson (1967). This may not be inevitable, however, since another study found that the reason for abortion, whether medical or psychological, was not an important factor in women's reactions (Simon et al. 1967). That study suggested, instead, that psychologically healthy women handled their abortions better than women with psychiatric difficulties, regardless of the indication for it. These contradictory findings highlight the importance of knowing each woman's particular situation and the need for new research.

Psychiatric History

Since most research on the psychiatric sequelae of abortion was done when the prevailing legal requirements for qualifying for an abortion would have led to an excess of subjects with preexisting psychiatric problems, it is difficult to determine the relative risk to women with and without previous psychiatric difficulties. (See Chapter 2.)

Interpersonal Relationships

Payne et al. (1976) found that women with negative relationships with their mothers, children, lovers, or husbands experienced significantly more anger, depression, and shame than women with positive relationships (see also Jansson 1965; Lask 1975; Shusterman 1979). They concluded that "1) a good relationship serves as a support and protection against depression resulting from loss and internal conflict; and 2) an unstable relationship frequently falls apart under the stress of an unwanted pregnancy, so that the woman must grieve the loss not only of the pregnancy, but of her lover as well. At the least, she goes through the experience without the father of the child" (p. 731).

Attitude Toward Pregnancy and Abortion

Women who are intensely ambivalent about pregnancy and abortion appear to suffer guilt and depression in the early postabortion period (Ashton 1980; Friedman et al. 1974; Lask 1975; Payne et al. 1976). Ambivalence is more likely when the pregnancy is desired. Women who do not want to become pregnant and who therefore use more effective means of birth control may have fewer emotional difficulties (Payne et al. 1976). But women who want to continue a pregnancy and are pressured into terminating it by family or physician (Niswander and Patterson 1967; Patt et al. 1969; Whittington 1970) or who do so to please a spouse or lover (Pasnau 1972) may have unfavorable outcomes.

Circumstances Surrounding Abortion

Pasnau (1972) described the case of a young woman admitted for a second-trimester saline abortion who was placed on the obstetric ward with newborn infants and mothers, treated by staff with irritation and disdain, and considered a "second-class citizen." This woman became severely depressed and suicidal. He wrote, "Negative and hostile attitudes on the part of hospital personnel and inadequate counseling and consideration for the patient's emotional state could be related directly to the incidence of postabortion guilt, remorse, and depression" (p. 255).

Issues in Treating Abortion-Related Problems

Mental health professionals not only evaluate and treat women who have been referred for treatment of psychiatric difficulties related to an abortion, they also may find themselves working with women who are already engaged in psychotherapy when they become pregnant. Therapy provides an opportunity to explore feelings about the pregnancy and to decide whether to maintain the pregnancy or seek an abortion. A woman who is considering terminating a pregnancy for any reason is experiencing a crisis in her life. Under pressure of time, she must make a decision that will affect her now and in the future and that may evoke unresolved feelings about herself and her significant past and present relationships. The therapist should convey to the woman concern and empathy for the turmoil she may be experiencing and provide support as necessary, perhaps through extra sessions, telephone conversations, or meetings with her partner or family. The therapist should help her explore her feelings and wishes so that she can make a truly free decision. Some women may need particular help containing their feelings so that they may make a rational decision; the therapist may need to examine with them the sources of their panic— perhaps pressure from others to choose a particular course—and provide clarification of distorted ideas and misperceptions. Other women may need help in recognizing the range of feelings that the pregnancy has elicited and support in working them through. The crisis may be especially intense for women who typically have trouble making decisions and for women who are intensely ambivalent or who are under pressure to choose a particular course. It may be more helpful to formulate the dilemma as "Do I have this child or not?" than as "Do I have an abortion or not?" (See Chapter 7.)

Other abortion-related issues may emerge during ongoing psychotherapy. Memories of a pregnancy that was terminated many years earlier may arise spontaneously; feelings about the abortion will become an important aspect of that phase of the therapy (see the case study of Anna T.). Issues related to a past abortion may surface at the time of a later pregnancy. Women who had an abortion when they were young and who encounter infertility problems at a time when they want to have a child may feel regret and anger in recalling the abortion. Unconscious feelings related to an abortion may provide the motivation for a woman to enter psychotherapy (see the case study of Susan L.), and these may emerge only by listening for such material in the patient's associations.

Mental health professionals may experience various countertransference reactions to a woman who is trying to decide about abortion or to the feelings she expresses about a past abortion. These reactions reflect the therapist's own religious, moral, and social beliefs; personal experiences; and the social and legal climate of the time. Therapists should monitor their emotional responses and, when they interfere with maintaining a dispassionate and therapeutic stance that allows the woman to know her own feelings and make her own free decision, should make every effort to understand the source of these responses and contain them. Consultation with a supervisor may be indicated if self-analysis is ineffective.

Clinical experience suggests that many women have an emotional response to abortion, but typically it is mild and short-lived. More pronounced reactions are generally the result of a complex set of factors and may be explained by the circumstances surrounding the pregnancy, the life stage and particular situation of the woman, the nature of the relationship between the woman and her partner, the woman's personality and psychodynamic history, and the values of her family and community. Psychotherapy should address the particular meaning that the pregnancy and abortion have for a woman and help her confront painful affects and unresolved conflicts. In many cases, distress related to an abortion comes not from the abortion but from long-standing issues and old losses that may be usefully dealt with in long-term psychotherapy. In other cases, support during the time of emotional distress and throughout the natural process of resolution may be all that is needed. In all cases, it is important to appreciate that pregnancy and abortion represent life crises that provide the opportunity for personal growth and greater self-awareness.

References

American Psychiatric Association: Position Statement on abortion. Am J Psychiatry 126:1554, 1970

Ashton JR: The psychosocial outcome of induced abortion. Br J Obstet Gynaecol 87:1115–1122, 1980

Barnes AB, Cohen E, Stoeckle JD, et al: Therapeutic abortion: medical and social sequels. Ann Intern Med 75:881–886, 1971

Brody H, Meikle S, Gerritse R: Therapeutic abortion: a prospective study. Am J Obstet Gynecol 109:347–353, 1971

Cavenar JO, Maltbie AA, Sullivan JL: Aftermath of abortion. Bull Menninger Clin 42:433–438, 1978

Ewing JA, Rouse BA: Therapeutic abortion and a prior psychiatric history. Am J Psychiatry 130:37–40, 1973

Ford C, Atkinson R, Bragonier J: Therapeutic abortion: who needs a psychiatrist? Obstet Gynecol 38:206–213, 1971a

Ford C, Castelnuovo-Tedesco P, Long K: Is abortion a therapeutic procedure in psychiatry? JAMA 218:1173–1178, 1971b

Friedman CM, Greenspan R, Mittleman F: The decision-making process and the outcome of therapeutic abortion. Am J Psychiatry 131:1332–1337, 1974

Gilligan C: In a Different Voice. Cambridge, MA, Harvard University Press, 1982

Greenglass ER: Therapeutic abortion and psychiatric disturbance in Canadian women. Can Psychiatr Assoc J 21:453–460, 1976

Group for the Advancement of Psychiatry: The Right to Abortion: A Psychiatric View. New York, Group for the Advancement of Psychiatry, 1969

Illsley R, Hall MH: Psychosocial aspects of abortion. Bull WORLD Health Organ 52:83–106, 1976

Jacobs D, Garcia CR, Rickels K, et al: A prospective study on the psychological effects of therapeutic abortion. Compr Psychiatry 15:423–434, 1974

Jansson B: Mental disorders after abortion. Acta Psychiatr Scand 41:87–110, 1965

Kent I, Breenwood RC, Loeken J, et al: Emotional sequelae of elective abortion. Br Columbia Med J 20:118–119, 1978

Kretzschmar RM, Norris AS: Psychiatric implications of therapeutic abortion. Am J Obstet Gynecol 98:368–373, 1967

Lask B: Short-term psychiatric sequelae to therapeutic termination of pregnancy. Br J Psychiatry 126:173–177, 1975

Marder L: Psychiatric experience with a liberalized therapeutic abortion law. Am J Psychiatry 126:1230–1236, 1970

Margolis AJ, Davison LA, Hanson KH, et al: Therapeutic abortion follow-up study. Am J Obstet Gynecol 110:243–249, 1971

Ney PG, Wickett AR: Mental health and abortion: review and analysis. Psychiatr J Univ Ottawa 14:506–516, 1989

Niswander KR, Patterson RJ: Psychologic reaction to therapeutic abortion, I: subjective patient response. Obstet Gynecol 29:702–706, 1967

Osofsky JD, Osofsky HJ, Rajan R, et al: Psychologic effects of legal abortion. Clin Obstet Gynecol 14:215–234, 1971

Pasnau RO: Psychiatric complications of therapeutic abortion. Obstet Gynecol 40:252–256, 1972

Patt SL, Rappaport RG, Barglow P: Follow-up of therapeutic abortion. Arch Gen Psychiatry 20:408–414, 1969

Payne EC, Kravitz AR, Notman MT, et al: Outcome following therapeutic abortion. Arch Gen Psychiatry 33:725–733, 1976

Roe v. Wade, 410 U.S. 113 (1973)

Shusterman LR: Predicting the psychological consequences of abortion. Soc Sci Med 13A:683–689, 1979

Simon NM, Senturia AG, Rothman D: Psychiatric illness following therapeutic abortion. Am J Psychiatry 124:59–65, 1967

Whittington HG: Evaluation of therapeutic abortion as an element of preventive psychiatry. Am J Psychiatry 126:1224–1229, 1970

Chapter 9

Issues for Staff Involved With Abortion

Miriam B. Rosenthal, M.D.
Florence R. Young, R.N., M.S.N.

There is a paucity of published studies on psychological issues faced by professional staffs involved in providing abortion services. The available literature and our observations indicate considerable variation in attitudes and feelings about abortion on the part of staff members. Although the differences cannot be empirically quantified or tested, we believe it is possible to make some valid generalizations while providing examples from our experience.

Valid generalizations may be made regarding practices of clinicians who represent different religious, cultural, and socioeconomic backgrounds. Likewise, generalizable differences can be observed between physicians and nurses and between nurses and social workers. It is desirable to consider these differences because they influence the character of the abortion experience for the gravida and its sequelae for her.

The environment in which abortions are currently provided in the United States is a source of conflict for some of those involved in abortion services. Abortions done in freestanding clinics have been the primary targets of activists in the so-called right-to-life movement. Staff members in these clinics often work with these activists picketing and shouting, impeding patient and staff access to the clinic. On the other hand, staff members

Many thanks go to Dr. Mary Mahowald, professor of bioethics, for her help in the preparation of the manuscript for this chapter.

working with abortion patients in a hospital setting have not generally been exposed to this kind of stress and may be involved with proportionately fewer abortion patients than staff members in freestanding clinics.

Historical Aspects

To understand better the present environment in which abortion services are provided in the United States, it is necessary to review briefly the history of abortion in this country. The medicalization of abortion procedures is recent, occurring in the latter half of the nineteenth century, when a movement was begun by American physicians to restrict access to abortion by making themselves gatekeepers. This movement was part of an effort at the time to provide better health care for women; to decrease maternal morbidity and mortality, by controlling where and when abortions were done; and to ensure that practitioners were adequately trained. Professionalism required increased knowledge and skills on the part of abortion providers (Imber 1986; Luker 1984; Rossi and Sitaraman 1988). This movement was led by members of the newly created American Medical Association. Most physicians of the period were white middle- and upper-class men who were willing to provide abortion services for women of their own social class who were "in trouble" (Luker 1984). They had strict criteria for providing abortions, and these criteria were often dictated by their own attitudes and morality. Some would only provide abortions if a mother's life was threatened by a medical condition. Others believed that quality-of-life issues were important and provided abortions for social or economic reasons (Luker 1984). In 1933, Abraham Rongy, a gynecologist, wrote a book advocating abortion when pregnancy was "illegitimate," when it occurred during a husband's desertion, or when it occurred during widowhood. He was widely criticized for these views.

Gradually, it became clear that the kind of abortion services available in any given community were determined by the ideas, values, morality, and opinions of the doctors practicing there (Imber 1986; Petchesky 1985). Although anecdotal reports existed, there were no surveys of physician attitudes before 1960. Abortions done for medical reasons were done quietly and considered acceptable, whereas those done for social, economic, or other reasons were considered criminal and often done by "abortionists," a pejorative term. Criminal abortion persisted because legal abortion was costly, difficult to obtain, and hard to get reliable information about. Fertility control was considered a very private matter and not to be discussed publicly. Marriage was viewed as the remedy for unwanted pregnancy in single women. Many abortions were done on married women, but the exact incidence is unknown. Mortality rates were not carefully recorded for single or married women. The Kinsey (1953) report showed that one of every four married women interviewed had had an abortion. Because of underreporting, the incidence is probably greater than the Kinsey data indicated.

Obstetricians and Gynecologists

Physicians most involved in providing abortions have been those who look after the health of women—obstetricians and gynecologists. Most obstetricians and gynecologists believe that they enter this field because they wish to preserve maternal and fetal life. If abortion was seen as therapeutic and was part of the overall care of mothers and infants, it was better accepted than if it was perceived as purely elective (Imber 1986). In addition to that philosophy, other factors affecting doctors' practices were and are the societal climate regarding abortion, its legality, public opinion, religion, education, and doctors' family situation, especially experiences with infertility or with children who have genetic abnormalities. Some physicians have basic moral objections to abortion, and others find the procedures emotionally distasteful and are repelled by the idea of doing them, although abortion itself is acceptable as a procedure—especially if it is therapeutic. Abortions done after long periods of infertility or for sex selection have been especially disturbing. Doctors still believe that they should have the right to participate or not, as do other health care workers.

Today, residents in obstetrics and gynecology training in the United States are expected to know how to perform an abortion or to refer patients to facilities where they are done, even if they are not willing to do them. The manual *Educational Objectives for Residents in Obstetrics and Gynecology* (Committee on Residency Education in Obstetrics and Gynecology 1984) states that a major objective for all of those who will practice this specialty is that they have the skill to perform an abortion and the ability to understand the counseling needs of a pregnant woman who requests one. For example, a trainee is asked to consider the case of a woman who is 9 weeks pregnant and requests an abortion. The trainee is expected to describe how arrangements should be made for such a patient to receive the appropriate care in a safe and experienced facility. Whether or not the trainee is prepared to perform the procedure, the response to the request should reflect adequate knowledge of acceptable alternatives.

Obstetricians and gynecologists today believe that they should perform abortions because the procedure requires considerable technical skill. They believe, as did their predecessors, that although they should have the control, no one should be forced to perform an abortion who does not wish to do so. This leads to some difficulties in training programs: some require all residents to perform abortions, others make abortions optional, and some forbid abortions entirely. Religion seems to be the most powerful predictor of whether obstetricians and gynecologists provide abortion services. One study shows that 85% of Roman Catholic physicians, 28% of Protestant doctors, and 9% of Jewish doctors do not perform abortions (Nathanson and Becker 1980). Most doctors who perform abortions believe that the procedure should be available, but with some restrictions regarding where it may be done, by whom, and the duration of gestation. Most doctors have fewer problems with first-trimester abortions than with second-trimester abortions. Some who strongly support a woman's right to abortion decline to perform them because they find them emotionally difficult; some who willingly perform abortions by indirect methods, such as prostaglandin or saline infusion, refuse to use direct methods, such as dilation and evacuation.

Our conversations with older obstetricians who provide abortions raised memories of great concern in the days before the legalization of abortion in 1973, when women came to the emergency rooms of hospitals very ill with infection or hemorrhage from complications of abortions done in squalid conditions by untrained individuals for considerable profit. Younger doctors take abortion practices more in stride, often wanting women to have that choice, even if they do not wish to perform them themselves.

A survey of gynecologists in Great Britain (Savage and Francone 1989) found that 75% of gynecologists believe that women have the right to decide about their pregnancies with their doctors and that the 1967 Abortion Act worked satisfactorily.

Residents in obstetrics, gynecology, and family medicine often admit that they have conflicting feelings about abortion procedures. Like some of their faculty supervisors, although they support reproductive choice, they dislike doing second-trimester abortions. They also have difficulty with women who are getting second and repeat abortions. Unlike the private practitioner who may know his or her patients well, residents frequently know little about the psychosocial situations of women for whom they care. Residents feel resentment toward patients who seem on the surface to take abortion lightly and have more sympathy toward women who look sad or serious (Mascovich et al. 1973). Other residents have considerably more empathy for women requesting abortion for conditions that threaten the mother's life, physical or psychological; for rape or incest; and for serious genetic defects. They have less sympathy for women who request abortion for economic hardship, for loss of a partner, or because they are overburdened with several other children. Many residents, however, become less judgmental during their training, such as a second-year resident in obstetrics who says that she chose a residency in which she would have the choice not to do abortions. She is Catholic and strongly opposed to abortion; however, her experiences are leading her to have a wider view, and now she is not sure what she will do when she has finished her training. Her attitude toward abortion seems to have changed by talking with women who have unwanted pregnancies because of rape or incest. She is trying to understand more of their lives and problems and the choices available to them.

Many physicians frankly tell us that they have more difficulty doing abortions on women whom they do not know, whereas others prefer to know nothing of the social situation of women, feeling that they are technicians with special expertise that they are willing to offer women who come to them for help.

Although physicians often believe that their attitudes and values regarding abortion are not apparent to their patients, especially in a general hospital setting, nurses who observe them do not always agree. Doctors may use rationalizations and intellectual defenses to explain their abortion practices, stating their belief that they were helping and working for the greater societal good. Doctors' views became more moderate as they continued to become more experienced and assisted at abortions. Interestingly, doctors with strong opposition came to be more in favor of reproductive choice for women, whereas those who were strong proponents of abortion rights became less enthusiastic. Kane et al. (1973) suggested the following procedures for obstetricians and gynecologists in hospitals who participate in abortion. Their participation should be voluntary. Medical leadership should be strongly supportive, with frequent group meetings to discuss problems and procedures. Abortion patients in general hospitals should be separated from obstetrical patients. The last suggestion is frequently not possible if only certain doctors do abortions and most referrals go to them. Kane also recommended training in counseling and psychosocial issues for obstetrical and gynecological residents to improve their skills in working with patients confronting reproductive issues.

Other Physicians

Different issues arise for physicians whose practice requires them to actually perform abortions and those who are involved in counseling or medical practice that might refer patients who need abortion for medical reasons. Doctors were asked, "Should abortion be available to any woman capable of giving legal consent upon her own request to a competent physician?" Most affirmative answers came from psychiatrists and allergists, and the fewest came from general practitioners, obstetricians, and general surgeons (Imber 1986). A problem with such surveys is that those who answer such broad questions may not approve of abortion under all circumstances but may approve of it under certain circumstances, or vice versa (Pratt 1976; Sheehan et al. 1980; Wolff et al. 1970).

In addition to differences in specialties, doctors are sensitive to their communities and culture in their practices. Doctors in urban areas are more likely to provide abortions than those in rural areas, where abortions are less well accepted. Those in the eastern United States, in New England, and on the Pacific Coast have more liberal attitudes than those in the Midwest or South. Those who disapprove of abortion tend to be more conservative and to have more conservative views about sex, homosexuality, and women's place in society (Granberg and Granberg 1980).

Since doctors are the chief limiting factor regarding the number of abortions done in hospitals where they practice, their overall reticence to perform abortions has caused a gradual shift of abortion procedures to freestanding clinics. This is especially true for first-trimester abortions that are done on women who have no special medical problems that would require hospital care. Medicaid will not pay for abortions unless they are done to protect the life of a mother. This has made it difficult for poor women on Medicaid, who receive most of their medical care in hospitals, to obtain abortions. Nonetheless, approximately 94% of women on Medicaid requesting abortions get them. In 1979, freestanding clinics provided 60% of all abortions. Doctors working in these clinics see themselves as performing a needed service. They do not have the same pressures as those in hospital settings who may be the object of disapproval from peers and other workers. Their pressures come from picketers and outside disapproval.

The increasingly strident presence of picketers from antiabortion groups has been unpleasant for those who have chosen to work in abortion clinics. In some cases, they have been not only harassed but endangered. The belief of the clinic personnel is that the men and women who have chosen to harass them have little knowledge of or empathy for women with a troubled pregnancy. It is interesting that staffs subjected to these abuses are growing increasingly angry and are choosing to become more active in the pro-choice movement.

The following personal observations provide an example of the pressures experienced by clinic personnel. As antiabortion picketers angrily screamed "murderers, murderers" outside a freestanding abortion clinic on a hot summer morning when the windows were open, the staff members grew increasingly angry as they tried to comfort a 12-year-old girl who had been raped, was pregnant, and had come for an abortion. Many of the staff members felt the need to believe that the protesters were irrational. The doctor ignored the protestors, denied their presence, and did his work.

There has been relatively little written about the effects on staff members of protesters creating scenes in front of abortion clinics. It has been very disruptive to the women coming for abortion who are already upset.

Psychiatrists

Before the U.S. Supreme Court *Roe v. Wade* (1973) decision, psychiatrists in many hospitals were required to write letters stating that a given woman would kill herself if she did not get an abortion. Many psychiatrists resented this role yet felt deeply that women have the right to choose. Since then, mental health professionals are more involved in counseling and the study of the psychological aspects of abortion. They have not found any increased psychiatric complications when comparing abortions with full-term births. The stress and coping of staff members is another useful area for study. Psychiatrists are concerned that if abortion becomes illegal again, they will be called on to be gatekeepers and to certify that an abortion is necessary to preserve a woman's mental health (Stotland 1989).

Nurses

Most of the nurses who go into maternity nursing do so because they enjoy working with pregnant women, caring for high-risk patients, or working in labor and delivery. When abortions are done in hospital settings, nurses may or may not have the choice of participating, since abortions done in hospitals are done by obstetric or gynecologic services. Most nurses consider themselves to be strong advocates for women's rights and are sensitive to the health issues of women. A national survey of students and faculty in schools of medicine, nursing, and social work indicated that nurses were the most conservative of all three groups in respect to abortion (Werley et al. 1973). At that time, abortion was just being made more available, and the observation may have since changed. Many nurses voice pro-choice sentiments, whereas others accept abortion only for special circumstances, such as rape, incest, congenital defects of major severity, or maternal disease that is life threatening. A study of nurses in Michigan and New York suggested that "increased exposure to easily available abortion procedures tends to promote a more favorable general attitude to abortion" (Allen et al. 1977).

Participation of nurses in hospital-based abortions has created certain conflicts for them. Nurses taking part in abortion procedures have rarely participated in the decision-making processes. They have conflicting feelings about a woman's right to reproductive choice versus their sense of frustration about participating in an abortion that is perceived as being done for economic or convenience reasons. Nurses assisting with second-trimester abortions feel especially ambivalent about patients who seem to have little understanding of the techniques and ask such questions as, What sex is it? May I have a picture? They may feel indignation when the physician is elsewhere and they are left to complete a second-trimester abortion after a saline or prostaglandin injection. In many hospitals, high-risk pregnancy patients are on the same floor with patients undergoing second-trimester abortions, and the same nurses are expected to care for all of them. In some instances, responsibilities for helping to maintain one pregnancy while endeavoring to terminate another lead to cognitive and moral dissonance. The same is true for doctors who care for abortion patients and high-risk pregnancy patients.

A head nurse who did not voice any objection to abortion but forgot to look in each morning on abortion patients illustrates how attitudes and behavior may be discordant and how staff members may deny their own feelings. Hospital-based nurses feel most supported by their peers who also participate, and they find the mutual support therapeutic. Some report that they do not discuss the abortion aspect of their work, feeling some shame and guilt about it.

Nurses working in freestanding clinics have chosen to work in such settings and participate in counseling and decision making. They feel more control, despite the presence of protesters in recent years. The nurses in these clinics are not judgmental and are supportive of the women for whom they provide care. They are similar to the nurses in the 1950s and 1960s who chose to work in family-planning clinics at a time when there was considerable public opposition to them. Group support is generally helpful to such individuals.

Burnout is a syndrome common to some workers who help in doing abortions. For doctors and nurses who are willing to participate, especially in second-trimester abortions, a feeling may grow of being overwhelmed and of doing the work for others who may not have ideologic objections but are lazy or biased, without a broader view of total health care for women. These staff members grow tired, feel put upon, and may become depressed. Mental health professionals should be part of this team, discussing cases and the feelings of the staff with them.

Social Workers

Social workers tend to have the same variety of attitudes as others in this field, but the major difference is that they are not called on to participate in the procedures. Social workers, by training, tend to have more liberal attitudes than physicians or nurses (Allen et al. 1977). Their training helps them to work with women trying to make difficult decisions so that these women may carry out the decisions themselves. It is usual for workers in maternity settings to have to deal with unwanted pregnancies in adolescents and adults. They have a deep understanding of the effects of poverty, violence, disruption, and mental illness on people's lives. They can be extremely helpful to doctors and nurses in telling them about the psychosocial situation that has brought a particular woman to make a particular decision. They lessen the anonymity of women in large urban hospitals and help individuals with decision making. They often feel frustrated at trying to get abortions for women who are poor and have few economic resources. Money needed for food and shelter may be used for obtaining an abortion. They struggle with their own conflicts, as do other health care workers (Hendershot and Grimm 1974).

Support Staff

Issues for support staff are frequently overlooked in hospital settings, and they may not even be clear to the staff members themselves. The following example was observed by us.

A secretary who worked in a maternity clinic in a large urban hospital serving mainly poor women denied having any bias about abortion. She was in charge of receiving all incoming calls for appointments. If a woman indicated she was interested in considering abortion, she was often scheduled weeks later than those requesting prenatal care. This led to women who might otherwise have had a first-trimester abortion requiring second-trimester abortions, which are more difficult for patients and more difficult to obtain. It is clear that this staff needed more help and support in working with abortion patients. Understanding more of her own attitude might have helped this woman to choose to work elsewhere or to alter her tendency to put off abortion patients.

Conclusion

No discussion of abortion is complete without consideration of the issues faced by medical practitioners and staff to whom a woman must turn when she desires to terminate a pregnancy. The environment in which she receives the counseling and care can have considerable influence on her physical and mental outcome. More needs to be heard from this group of people about the stress and gratification in their work.

References

Allen D, Reichdt P, Shea FP: Two measures of nurses' attitudes toward abortion as modified by experience. Med Care 15:849–857, 1977

Attitudes to Abortion. Br Med J 2:69, 1974

Committee on Residency Education in Obstetrics and Gynecology: Educational Objectives for Residents in Obstetrics and Gynecology, 3rd Edition. Committee on Residency Education in Obstetrics and Gynecology, 1984

Granberg D, Granberg B: Abortion attitudes, 1965–80: trends and determinants. Fam Plann Perspect 12:250–261, 1980

Hendershot G, Grimm J: Abortion attitudes among nurses and social workers. Am J Public Health 64:438–441, 1974

Imber J: Abortion and the Private Practice of Medicine. New Haven, CT, Yale University Press, 1986

Kane F, Feldman M, Jain S, et al: Emotional reactions in abortion services personnel. Arch Gen Psychiatry 28:409–411, 1973

Kinsey A: Sexual Behavior in the Human Female. Philadelphia, PA, WB Saunders, 1953

Luker K: Abortion and the politics of motherhood. Berkeley, CA, University of California Press, 1984

Mascovich P, Behrstock B, Minor D, et al: Attitudes of obstetric and gynecologic residents toward abortion. Calif Med 119:29–34, 1973

Nathanson C, Becker M: Obstetricians' attitudes and hospital abortion services. Fam Plann Perspect 12:26, 1980

Petchesky R: Abortion and Women's Choice. Boston, MA, Northeastern University Press, 1985, p 159

Pratt G: Connecticut physicians' attitudes toward abortion. Am J Public Health 66:288–290, 1976

Roe v. Wade, 410 U.S. 113 (1973)

Rongy A: Abortion: Legal or Illegal. New York, Vanguard, 1933

Rossi A, Sitaraman B: Abortion in context: historical trends and future changes. Fam Plann Perspect 20:273–281, 1988

Savage W, Francone C: Gynaecologists' attitudes to abortion. Lancet 2:1323–1324, 1989

Sheehan M, Munro J, Ryan J: Attitudes of medical practitioners towards abortion: a Queensland study. Australian Family Physician 9:565–570, 1980

Stotland N: Psychiatrists fear abortion decision will put profession in gatekeeper role. Psychiatric News, August 4, 1989

Werley H, Ager J, Rosen R, et al: Medicine, nursing, social work: professionals and birth control—student and faculty attitudes. Fam Plann Perspect 5:42, 1973

Wolff J, Nielson P, Schiller P: Therapeutic abortion: attitudes of medical personnel leading to complications in patient care. Am J Obstet Gynecol 110:730–733, 1970

Chapter 10

Male Experience of Elective Abortion: Psychoanalytic Perspectives

Arden Rothstein, Ph.D.

The aim of this chapter is to explore psychoanalytic perspectives on elective abortion with particular attention to the male partner's experience. A clinical interview study of the experience of men accompanying their partners to an abortion clinic after the decision to terminate a pregnancy is described. (Other facets of this study have been presented in Rothstein 1974, 1977a, 1977b, 1978.)

Rationale of the Study

This study would seem to be important from two interrelated perspectives. First, this event would be expected to have meaning to male partners as well as to women undergoing abortion. Knowledge about this subject would help guide clinical work with men who are currently considering or have previously considered elective abortion. In extension of the concept of normal developmental crises, one of my premises is that abortion may act as either a facilitator or a derailer of development, depending on factors such as the individual's ego organization and object relationships.

Second, given the frequency of elective abortion and the many significant psychological threads and meanings that a clinician might expect to accrue to this event, further investigation would be likely to contribute to developmental theory. Conceptualizations of development that are longitudinal and epigenetic in nature suggest that this, like any important life event, will not only influence but also be influenced by ongoing developmental processes. It was expected that in the case of these men, the process of abortion would be likely to influence the development of fatherliness and parenthood.

Conditions of the Study

Sixty males who accompanied their female partners to the abortion clinic of a large municipal teaching hospital were randomly selected from the clinic waiting area for clinical interviews. Forty interviews were structured (ranging from 45 to 90 minutes), and 20 were open-ended (from 90 to 135 minutes).

Review of the Literature

There has been little psychodynamic attention to women's responses to abortion (Pines 1982; Rosen 1970; Schaffer and Pine 1972; Shainess 1970; White 1970) and none to those of men. Indeed, only several publications of any orientation exist about men (Brahams 1987; Pitts 1988; Robbins 1984; Sarrel 1988; Walter 1970; WNBC-TV 1972). One unpublished study by WNBC-TV in New York in 1972 reported a large-scale opinion survey of men whose partners had not had abortions. Walter (1970) described a Kinsey group study that showed that only 4.2% of male partners had psychiatric sequelae. An abortion's psychodynamic meaning for those affected and for those who weathered the experience without symptomatology was not discussed.

This may be, in part, a natural consequence of the conditions of the event that do not readily lend themselves to collection of the intensive data with which psychoanalytically oriented therapists generally work. There is a brief period between definitive diagnosis of pregnancy and performance of the abortion procedure, which is itself simple and rapid in most cases. Therefore, relationships with hospital personnel are transient and follow-up contact is not routine. For multiple reasons, situational and psychological, this event fosters action rather than reflection. Nevertheless, as Schaffer and Pine (1972) found in a study of adolescent girls undergoing abortion, because of the crisis nature of the event, some people are unusually willing to discuss their experiences at this time if one only approaches them. It is commonly observed that rigid character defenses may be at least temporarily unavailable in the midst of the regression and anxiety that characterize a state of crisis (Bibring 1959; Bibring et al. 1961).

Clinical and Developmental Framework

The Theory of Developmental Crises

The psychoanalytic literature on developmental processes and crises offers several important perspectives on abortion. Of profound importance is A. Freud's (1965) appreciation of the irregular course of child development. Rather than following an ever-forward, uninterrupted path, normal development includes episodes of temporary regression. Other authors have extended this principle beyond childhood. It has been recognized that development is facilitated by an optimum degree of stress and gratification eventuating in growth and reorganization.

Awareness that crises do not necessarily have deleterious consequences has led psychoanalytically oriented researchers to study various crises. They have defined the issues they are likely to elicit—based on knowledge of the developmental stage of the patient and the symbolic meanings of the event—and explored the range of adaptive and maladaptive solutions. These include normal (psychological and psychophysiological) developmental crises and traumatic crises.

How might we view elective abortion? In one sense it is not a normal developmental process or stage but the interruption of one—pregnancy or parenthood. It is expected that some clinicians might, therefore, regard it as a trauma. It seems more accurate, however, to consider abortion along a continuum of developmental crises ranging from universal to elective, yet common. Universal developmental crises include those disturbances of psychic equilibrium that are an inevitable part of the development of the ego, object relations, and physiological maturation (e.g., rapprochement, toilet training, oedipal conflict, puberty, and climacterium). Crises that are optional (even though they may be psychologically determined) but so common as to approximate normal developmental crises include separation from the family upon entry into college, marriage, and parenthood. Less common but, nevertheless, too frequent in our society to be regarded as anomalous and rare traumata are elective events, such as divorce and abortion. As society changes, our concepts of psychopathology and trauma will subtly change. Like the normal developmental crises, elective abortion is experienced by many psychologically well-integrated people, and it has psychodynamic meanings that are closely related to these processes.

The Development of Fatherhood and Adolescence

Study of abortion is relevant to the interest increasingly shown in fatherhood and fatherliness (Benedek 1970; Cath et al. 1982, 1989; Lamb

1986). These are viewed as lifelong processes of development with genetic roots in the preoedipal and oedipal years. When a pregnancy occurs (even though it may not be carried to term), there are implications for the development of fatherliness.

There is a consensus in the analytic literature that the wish to have a child undergoes repression in adolescence. However, given the unexpected finding in this study that more than half (58.3%) of an unselected group of subjects were in one or another stage of adolescence—*middle, late,* or *post*-adolescence (Blos 1962)—it also became necessary to consider the impact of this experience on normal developmental issues of this stage of life. The issues and conflicts that are characteristic of adolescence are likely to be affected in some way by the experience of abortion. First, an abortion may reawaken impulses and fantasies that are normally repressed, possibly lending them a new and threatening reality (A. Freud 1958). Second, the event of a pregnancy and the subsequent termination of it directly touch on impulses and conflicts that are typically at the core of adolescence.

Let us briefly review them. The hallmarks of adolescence include object removal (Katan 1951), a second individuation (Blos 1962) culminating in a sense of identity in general and further consolidation of sexual identity in particular, and alteration of ego and superego organization in the face of reawakened pregenital and genital impulses combined with the new and more intense sexual impulses of puberty. These aspects of reorganization, accompanied by cognitive growth, also result in an adolescent's confrontation with the possibilities and limitations of his future existence.

Findings

The adaptation to abortion of each interview subject was considered in terms analogous to those employed by Kestenberg (1964) and Bibring (1959) in their discussions of menarche as a trigger mechanism for organization and pregnancy as a normal crisis. In the context of menarche, growth involved more mature thinking and increased organization of behavior and thought. Conflicts became more clearly delineated and, therefore, subject to reflection, and previous fantasy was differentiated from reality, resulting in improved reality testing. In Bibring's view, changes in self-image, movement toward appropriate identifications, and emotional investment in a child as a separate object suggested maturation. Kestenberg conceptualized lack of growth or disorganization as involving vague and disjointed communications and approaches to problem solving, and defensive denial or repression of information and observations with substitution of ideas stemming from individual pathology, which might further contribute to anxiety, depression, and disorganization of ego functions for mastery. Similarly, Bibring thought that loosening of normal defenses and appearance of primitive content indicate a pathological response; she also noted the possibility of major shifts in relationships and activities.

Abortion offered the possibility of growth in that it facilitated fantasying about being a partner, with related alterations in self-image and further consolidation of sexual identity. It also provided an opportunity for taking active control of the future, mastering stress in the present, and coping with other issues that became superimposed on and expressed through the abortion. Lack of growth in the case of abortion could be seen in weakening of usual defenses, vague thinking and communication about the prospect of parenthood, failure to confront directly the decision at hand, and a disorganized approach to problem solving. This often included defensive inattention to the events and facts of abortion with emergence of idiosyncratic, often primitive, ideas. These all served to minimize the effectiveness of ego controls over feelings of anxiety and depression.

At a time when a boy becomes physiologically capable of impregnation and experiences newly intensified sexual urges but has not yet found other than parental objects toward whom to direct these urges, repression of the wish to have a child is adaptive. The unplanned impregnation can be viewed as an attempt at removal of the incestuous object as the aim of sexual impulses. At the same time, this constitutes a failure (perhaps a return of the repressed) in that the adolescent, often unable to take full responsibility for deciding on and financing an abortion, seeks parental help; thus parental objects regain intimate contact with the adolescent's body and sexuality. For many adolescents, marked conflict over this was exemplified by distressed pleas that all information be kept confidential from parental objects, their own or those of their female partners. This made no logical sense, since inquiry revealed that parents almost always knew about the pregnancy. It did make psychological sense, however. Intense oedipal guilt was associated with the concrete proof of sexuality (pregnancy), often more so than with the abortion itself. Fearing loss of parental love and nurturance, the abortion unconsciously enabled eradication of this proof if no records remained.

Repression of the wish for a child also included previous fear and envy of the female who was perceived as dangerous, active, and powerful because of her childbearing capacities; these earlier fostered a feminine identification. Indeed, the exaggerated active stance of preadolescence has been described as an effort to ward off fantasied threats of feminine identification and fears of castration at the hands of women (Blos 1965). Having just successfully resolved these fears and conflicts, the adolescent who is faced with pregnancy and choices for abortion has to deal with similar fears again. At the same time, the ability to impregnate may reassure the adolescent of his intactness and potency and, since the abortion is performed on the female, fuel fears of her retaliatory rage.

At a time when other efforts at self-definition involve rebellion and independent activity, the tender (equated with passive) fantasies that a boy may have about a fetus or female partner can pose a further threat. Furthermore, earlier oedipal rivalrous fantasies of competing with father by giving a baby to mother may be both gratified and frustrated. Thoughts of proceeding with a pregnancy and giving mother the baby may be entertained. Yet the ultimate decision to terminate the pregnancy leaves the adolescent in a position of oedipal defeat.

It became clear that this need not be the exclusive response. The event of a pregnancy stimulated fantasies of being a father in which comparisons with one's own father, as well as with one's ego ideal of fatherhood, were implicit. These involved consideration of capacities as a caretaker and provider in the narrow sense of specifically parental responsibilities and in the broader sense of pleasure in relating to others in a nurturant fashion and effectively managing one's own affairs. In this way, abortion may influence the development of fatherliness. Effective management of the event might enhance a developing sense of competence and autonomy and foster identifications with others who are competent in managing difficult experiences. Conversely, it might impede this development. When fears of punishment, rejection, or other types of retribution for independent and potentially controversial action predominated over pleasure in fantasizing about and exercising personal choices, the impact was a regressive one and contributed to lowered self-esteem.

Since abortion is the termination of a potential life, concerns about aggression, guilt, and an expectation of blame for committing the act of abortion were anticipated. Surprising, however, was the variability of definitions of the agent and object of aggression. Oedipal and preoedipal guilt and fears of bodily threat in response to competitive strivings, rage, and sexuality were elicited to different degrees and with varying emphases, depending on the individual's history and dynamics. Although the males most often viewed themselves as harmful to their female partners, prospective children, or both, some of them experienced the female or her parents as the sole agent of aggression toward the fetus and her own body or other central aspects of self.

Finally, the need to decide whether to continue the pregnancy confronted some adolescents with limits and the definitive fact that their childhood was over. Alternatively, termination of the pregnancy could contribute to preservation of the childhood illusion of no limits.

Case Studies

Case studies are presented from two perspectives: 1) the degree of progressive versus regressive adaptation to abortion and 2) the psychological issues elicited and expressed by the unwanted pregnancy and the process of considering or experiencing abortion.

Mr. C: A Predominantly Progressive Experience of Abortion

Mr. C, a 23-year-old Puerto Rican man, accompanied his wife of the same age and background to an abortion clinic when she was approximately 12 weeks pregnant. Mr. C was in training to be a policeman, and Mrs. C was a housewife with a high school education and aspirations to be a nurse. The couple had been married for 5½ years, the marriage precipitated by the unplanned conception of their first child, now 5 years old. They continued to use unreliable contraceptive methods, resulting in a second unplanned pregnancy 2 years later, which was also carried to term.

Despite their formal marriage, the C's had not functioned as an independent couple. They were heavily dependent on Mrs. C's parents. They had experienced two separations, the first when Mr. C was sent to Vietnam and the second, a year after their reunion, which was attributed to marital conflict. When Mr. C refused Mrs. C's demand to move to Puerto Rico where her parents had recently relocated, she took off in protest with their children to live with her parents. At the time of the clinic visit, the couple had been reunited only 3 weeks. Mrs. C discovered that she was pregnant upon her arrival in Puerto Rico several weeks before and notified Mr. C indirectly through family members.

The predominant themes of Mr. C's interview were his need to assert control over others (and over his own life), his pleasure at a newly acquired sense of commitment to his goals, and his competence and self-reliance as a caretaker and provider. The importance of being in control stemmed from past and present events. According to Mr. C, his wife had recently deserted him because he would not accommodate her wishes. He refused to move to Puerto Rico, at least at the specific time she designated. He desired to move only after completing his professional training. He felt hurt and enraged by his wife's abandonment.

Such a loss of honor and prestige was also experienced by Mr. C earlier in life, at the time of his wife's first pregnancy. He was then confronted with his sensed inability, at the age of 17, to stand up to his wife's father, who disapproved of him as a husband for his daughter and demanded an abortion. Mr. C turned to his own father to aid him in taking a firm stance against this plan. He felt that were it not for his father, he would have been powerless: "I told my father because I couldn't stop him myself." Mr. C's pervasive feeling was that he had not determined his own life choices; things had happened to him rather than his making them happen. On the occasion of his wife's third pregnancy, it became important to him to have a child electively, instead of by accident. He noted that once his (and perhaps his wife's) education was completed, "We got to have one more baby, one we planned, ourselves, one we talk about."

Until the return of his wife and children and the discovery of the pregnancy and subsequent plans for abortion, Mr. C seemed to have a disappointing view of himself as a father and husband: "Before I wasn't a very good father." He fell far short of his ego ideal of fatherhood, based on perceptions of his own father. At the same time, Mr. C wished to have more for himself.

Overall, the abortion seemed to have an organizing effect on Mr. C. This great event occurred at a critical point in his life and had a good fit with important genetic and developmental issues and conflicts. At the time of the abortion, although 23 years old and married for 5 years with two children, Mr. C had just begun to develop the integrating professional and personal goals and commitments of late adolescence. His marriage was in jeopardy, and he experienced a severe narcissistic injury at the hands of his wife. After an initially symptomatic response of depression and passivity, he mobilized himself to face the prospect of abortion.

The abortion seemed to serve multiple functions for him. He could exercise control over and express rage toward his wife who had just abandoned him to assert her will. Of equal importance was Mr. C's ability, with enhanced capacities and financial means, to manage this third unplanned pregnancy quite differently from the previous two. Rather than recapitulate the sense of humiliation he felt in being overpowered by his wife's father and childishly needy of his own father, he was now afforded a more satisfactory resolution. Mr. C carefully researched the array of available abortion services and understood the procedure with remarkable clarity. Mr. C experienced a sense of taking active hold of the future (in not having another birth happen to him) and found the pleasure of commitment in accepting limits.

His self-esteem was simultaneously enhanced as he better realized his ego ideal of fatherhood. Mr. C was surprised and greatly reassured to discover that he was capable of many of the qualities he so revered in his father and of advancing himself in his career. "Five years ago," he noted, "I would have left my wife or told her to get out. I would not have carried out these responsibilities." He now felt himself to be competent, nurturant, loyal, firm but gentle, and self-sacrificing yet self-respecting. He was able to parent his children, as well as his wife (in the situation of abortion), with new dedication. He felt a duty to delay (but not surrender) the completion of his education because of financial responsibilities. The feminine associations of such behavior had previously threatened his machismo-invested self-representation. At the time of the abortion, Mr. C was more accepting of his feminine identifications. He joked about his fantasies of men becoming pregnant sometime in the future and likened his transient loss of appetite to morning sickness.

This is not to suggest that Mr. C's conflicts about his passive wishes and tendencies were resolved. His exaggerated emphasis on taking care of the abortion and his family single-handedly belied his intense need to be a particular kind of man. Yet he was surprisingly aware of his own vulnerabilities and self-doubts; able to admit to me, a woman, how helpful our interview was to him in that he could unburden his feelings; and capable of acknowledging his potential need for psychiatric consultation.

Mr. D: A Predominantly Regressive Experience of Abortion

The case of Mr. D illustrates abortion as a disorganizing crisis. Mr. D, a 25-year-old white Roman Catholic man, accompanied his 20-year-old white Roman Catholic girlfriend to an abortion clinic 1½ weeks after they definitively confirmed her pregnancy. She was in her 12th week of pregnancy at the time of abortion. This was the first pregnancy for both partners. They had dated each other steadily for 2 years but had only recently started sexual relations. The man claimed to have prior sexual experience. His girlfriend, however, was reportedly a virgin until their recent involvement. The couple had no plans for marriage and no previous marital history. Mr. D, a college graduate, lived with his parents and was enrolled in several additional courses requisite for his application to medical school. This was a career plan only recently formulated. Throughout college, Mr. D felt aimless, although his grades were excellent. His girlfriend, a college sophomore, resided with her parents.

Mr. D expressed several closely related themes in the course of his interview. Most central was his shame related to a sense of having lost his capacity for autonomous and effective functioning by getting into this predicament. He felt he had acted unwisely and irresponsibly in impregnating his girlfriend, for which he feared punishment and possible rejection. This situation had particular importance for Mr. D in that it threatened to recapitulate his older brother's experience of "falling into the trap" of marrying his girlfriend because she became pregnant. In so doing he had also fallen out of grace with his parents, who were disparaging of the marriage. For Mr. D, the current illegitimate pregnancy raised the specter of losing his parents' admiration and his victory over his brother. At the same time, the pregnancy might have been symptomatic of Mr. D's conflicts over success, particularly in relation to his brother. Mr. D feared loss of his parents' love and their financial assistance in response to the pregnancy. Guilt over his parents' or his girlfriend's parents' discovery that he and his girlfriend engaged in sexual relations was an issue to Mr. D but not central to his conscious experience of abortion. Other intense fears of punishment may have been displaced expressions of guilt: that his girlfriend's mother (who had a heart condition) would die if she learned of the abortion ("and I would always have that on my conscience") or that his girlfriend might die of hemorrhaging. The latter fears may also have been expressions of rage at his girlfriend for setting the "trap" (of pregnancy) and part of the overwhelming sense of panic and helplessness that most notably characterized him. At the same time, the pregnancy might have been symptomatic of Mr. D's conflicts over success, particularly in relation to his brother.

The interview with Mr. D was marked by extreme anxiety and an inability to come to terms with its determinants: "I'm blank now . . . tomorrow I'll analyze it," he noted. His handling of the abortion and of contraception was in keeping with his tendency to avoidance or blocking in the face of overwhelming anxiety and his strong investment in not appearing dumb at all costs. Although Mr. D claimed to have used contraception with previous girlfriends, in this case he left the matter to his girlfriend, with no assurance that she took care of it. He engaged in repeated self-recrimination for this.

There was a similar failure to confront suggestions that his girlfriend was pregnant, which were evident well before 12 weeks. Mr. D noted that he had "deluded" himself into believing "it wouldn't happen" and inventing unlikely explanations to account for her missed menstrual periods. Vagueness and defensive inattention also characterized Mr. D's knowledge of the events and facts of the abortion procedure. This was particularly noteworthy, given that he was a premedical student and had many friends who were medical students or interns. He had consulted with them about the quality of care at the hospital in which the abortion was to be performed but not about the nature of the procedure. Mr. D also avoided discussion of the decision for abortion with his girlfriend and did not engage in fantasying about parenthood. He explained that he and his girlfriend agreed about the abortion, making further communication about it unnecessary.

The inaccessibility of Mr. D's feelings and fantasies, even to himself, was remarkable. His conscious experience was of intense, diffuse anxiety and regressive wishes. He angrily demanded special attention from the clinic staff, whom he criticized for their unemotional qualities:

I don't want to just hear she comes in and the procedure takes so long. . . . I wanted to hear this big elaborate story of how the doctor is here all the time, reassurance . . . to be sure nothing would go wrong. . . . How about me? Do they have something for me to lay on while I die? . . . I'm a wreck. . . .

It is noteworthy that Mr. D was gradually able to make some use of the interview to aid him in exploring the sources of his anxiety and ultimately in calming down. In the context of discussion with a person he would not see again, his admission of what he did not know was facilitated. Furthermore, as he was furnished facts and encouraged to confront his own concerns, his anxiety was diminished to some degree.

The abortion might have offered Mr. D a means of undoing his sense of stupidity and ineffectiveness, in preventing the recapitulation of his brother's "weak" mistake, and, therefore, in bolstering his self-esteem. Mr. D, instead, experienced himself as particularly dumb and helpless in the handling of the abortion, which further lowered his self-esteem. Mr. D had a regressive reaction, characterized by overwhelming anxiety, reliance on ineffective defenses, and increased dependency needs.

Implications for Clinical Practice

The findings of this exploratory study have implications for the clinical needs of male partners of women having abortions, at the time of the abortion procedure and when they later present themselves for psychotherapy and report a history of abortion.

Several findings and observations suggest that male partners should be allowed and encouraged to be more active participants in the abortion process:

1. They were involved in, but not overwhelmed by, the abortion.
2. They clearly expressed more interest in participation than was being tapped. Furthermore, greater interest was elicited as they became better informed.
3. Few knew about abortion and some had distorted ideas.
4. They experienced relief with knowledge.
5. They were inhibited in revealing fear and guilt feelings about the abortion, but with further exploration they seemed to feel freer to do so. Many of them had not discussed the abortion with people other than their partners.
6. They felt that they offered (and, in fact, might have offered) significant support to their partners, with whom they often had stable and long-standing relationships.
7. An active caretaking role may help some to defend against regressive tendencies and to better realize their parental ego ideals.

Without purporting to develop a detailed health program for these men, several suggestions will be made about some of the directions such a program might take. In large measure these derive from subjects' direct statements; others were stimulated by the needs they evidenced. In particular, the men seemed to require information about contraception and abortion and an opportunity to express their feelings about abortion and related matters.

Men in this study exhibited a striking lack of knowledge about abortion. Few men demonstrated an accurate or complete understanding of how abortions are performed. Furthermore, their incorrect or distorted ideas often reflected personal needs or wishes. Again, a short, straightforward explanation of the two major abortion procedures might greatly aid these men in detoxifying their often fantastic ideas. This is not to suggest that distortions will be relinquished by all men. The feelings and impulses that they have expressed will persist; however, these feelings and impulses may become more available for exploration or be more easily kept under control once the real nature of the abortion procedure is spelled out.

In addition to the feelings based on unconscious conflicts (e.g., those expressed in fantasies about how abortions are performed), male partners verbalized, more or less reluctantly, many other concerns elicited by the abortion. These included actual or anticipated conflicts with partners or parents over the decision for abortion, guilt about electing to terminate a life, anxiety about the psychological or physical effect of abortion on partners, and financial considerations. It seems important to offer these men an opportunity to discuss and resolve some of their anxieties related to abortion in one of three modalities: individual discussions with clinic mental health workers, joint interviews with their partners and mental health workers, and discussion groups with other men at which a clinic staff member is present.

Although a best approach to the clinical needs of men whose partners have elective abortions has not yet been identified, it seems clear that the extant system is unsatisfactory. It either ignores the needs of these men entirely or assumes that information is disseminated to them through their partners. Past research (Komarovsky 1962; Ostrum 1972) and the current study suggest that this latter assumption is fallacious. Of course, in devising new services, the exigencies of time and money must be recognized. At least two of these suggestions do not involve significant additional expenditures: including men when information is imparted to their partners and dispersing information in the form of pamphlets or videotapes. Other suggestions (e.g., individual educational sessions with men and opportunities to explore feelings) would necessitate additional personnel or at least reallocation of the time of those already on staff.

The impact on women of men's greater knowledge about and participation in aspects of the abortion process has not been a subject of this study; the needs of male partners have been discussed, for the most part, in isolation from those of their partners. This impact on women remains to be explored. It seems unlikely, however, that men who are interested in being involved, and who seemed to gain from the minimal participation permitted by this study, could be anything but additionally and meaningfully supportive of their partners.

There are probably few clinicians today whose practice does not include some mention of abortion. When such a history is reported, several clinical findings of this study should be kept in mind. For most men, the abortion was a significant experience but not an overwhelming or disorganizing one. A wide variety of issues, instead of a limited number of common themes, was elicited by this experience and seemed to be contingent on personal dynamics and histories rather than demographic features. Most of the men whose partners had abortions were far from indifferent to the idea of parenthood; instead, they were strongly invested in realizing their ego ideals of fatherhood, although only a minority were actively engaged in considering this prospect for the near future. The abortion was handled adequately by most men and seemed to provide an opportunity for adaptive organization or relief for those who were able to consciously experience and weigh feelings and needs and to maintain self-esteem by performing as supportive partners and making workable plans.

The many adolescents found in this study sample suggest that the incidence of adult patients presenting themselves for psychoanalytically oriented psychotherapy who will have experienced or considered an abortion as adolescents is likely to increase. At least two important implications exist, one for treatment of adolescents and adults and the other for treatment of adults only. First, when a history of abortion emerges, whether for an adolescent or adult patient, awareness of this event as a possible derailer or organizer of development should be heightened, given that regression and disequilibrium are normative at this stage. Questions about the residua of this event and its effect on character development should be raised.

Second, increased knowledge of the dynamic meanings and impact of this event may aid in some of the often-noted difficulties in reconstructing adolescent experience in an affective-laden way (A. Freud 1958). Abortion may serve as a nodal point around which other elicited memories may revolve, given the multiple developmental trends that may be tapped.

Suggestions for Future Research

Follow-up interviews should be arranged after 6 months or more, to see how an abortion is resolved and integrated and, more specifically, whether its apparently minor disruptive impact (or its organizing effect) at the time of acute crisis is maintained. There should be individual interviews with male partners and then joint interviews with both partners at the time of an abortion to gain a better picture of the extent to which each partner corroborates the feelings of the other or the extent to which projection is used to resolve ambivalent feelings. There should be in-depth exploration of women's feelings about involving their partners in abortion to a greater extent. There should be a more systematic assessment of the effect of instruction or intervention with men whose partners are undergoing abortions. Men who do not accompany their partners should be studied to see whether they ought to be encouraged to participate.

In summary, there is no doubt that some men are concerned about their partners' abortions, that they express interest in greater participation, and that they benefit from that participation. The effects of such involvement at the time of an abortion, its lasting impact, and the value of instituting policies to address partners' needs should be studied.

References

Benedek T: Fatherhood and providing, in Parenthood: Its Psychology and Psychopathology. Edited by Anthony EJ, Benedek T. Boston, MA, Little, Brown, 1970, pp 167–183

Bibring G: Some considerations of the psychological processes in pregnancy. Psychoanal Study Child 14:113–121, 1959

Bibring G, Dwyer T, Huntington D, et al: A study of the psychological processes in pregnancy. Psychoanal Study Child 16:9–72, 1961

Blos P: On Adolescence. New York, Free Press, 1962

Blos P: The initial stage of male adolescence. Psychoanal Study Child 20:145–164, 1965

Brahams D: An action by putative father and unborn fetus to prevent termination. Lancet 1:576–577, 1987

Cath S, Gurwitt A, Ross JM (eds): Father and Child. Boston, MA, Little, Brown, 1982

Cath S, Gurwitt A, Gunsberg L (eds): Fathers and Their Families. Hillsdale, NJ, Analytic Press, 1989

Freud A: Adolescence. Psychoanal Study Child 13:255–278, 1958

Freud A: Normality and Pathology in Childhood. New York, International Universities Press, 1965

Katan A: The role of displacement in agoraphobia. Int J Psychoanal 32:41–50, 1951

Kestenberg JS: Menarche, in Adolescents. Edited by Lorand S, Schneer HI. New York, Harper & Row, 1964, pp 19–50

Komarovsky M: Blue Collar Marriage. New York, Random House, 1962

Lamb ME (ed): The Father's Role. New York, John Wiley, 1986

Ostrum AE: Psychological factors influencing women's choice of childbirth procedure. Unpublished doctoral dissertation, Columbia University, New York, 1972

Pines D: The relevance of early psychic development to pregnancy and abortion. Int J Psychoanal 63:311–319, 1982

Pitts AG: Male abortion counseling: prevention of repeat abortions through male counseling. Conn Med 52:209–210, 1988

Robbins JM: Out-of-wedlock abortion and delivery: the importance of the male partner. Social Problem 31:334–350, 1984

Rosen H: Abortion and psychiatry: the effect of abortion upon psychic equilibrium and vice versa (panel report), in Abortion in a Changing World, Vol 2. Edited by Hall RE. New York, Columbia University Press, 1970, pp 53–68

Rothstein A: The "would-have-been-father": a descriptive study of men accompanying their partners to an abortion clinic. Unpublished doctoral dissertation, Columbia University Teachers College, New York, 1974

Rothstein A: Abortion: a dyadic perspective. Am J Orthopsychiatry 47:111–118, 1977a

Rothstein A: Men's reactions to their partners' elective abortions. Am J Obstet Gynecol 128:831–837, 1977b

Rothstein A: Adolescent males, fatherhood, and abortion. J Youth Adol 7:203–214, 1978

Sarrel PM: Male abortion counseling. Conn Med 52:244, 1988

Schaffer C, Pine F: Pregnancy, abortion, and the developmental tasks of adolescence. J Am Acad Child Psychiatry 11:511–546, 1972

Shainess N (panelist): Abortion and psychiatry: the effect of abortion upon psychic equilibrium and vice versa, in Abortion in a Changing World. Edited by Hall RE. New York, Columbia University Press, 1970, pp 134–175

Walter GS: Psychologic and emotional consequences of elective abortion: a review. Obstet Gynecol 36:482–491, 1970

White RA (panelist): Abortion and psychiatry: the effect of abortion upon psychic equilibrium and vice versa, in Abortion in a Changing World. Edited by Hall RE. New York, Columbia University Press, 1970, p 238

WNBC-TV: Population attitudes study. Unpublished survey, New York, 1972

Chapter 11

Second-Trimester Abortion

Shaila Misri, M.D., F.R.C.P.(C)
Eileen Anderson, R.N., B.Sc.N., M.Ed.

Feelings associated with second-trimester abortion may be particularly intense. Compared to the first trimester, the fetus is more developed; many of the fetal characteristics resemble those of a full-term infant; and the woman may feel fetal movement and begin to identify the fetus as a child.

Psychiatrists are seldom involved in the decision making surrounding second-trimester abortions, and a lack of definitive research impedes recommendations concerning such involvement. Most abortion research has been limited to case studies, has included first-trimester abortion in the findings, or has contained other methodological flaws (Adler 1980; Hall et al. 1987). It has also relied mainly on self-report measures with questionable results (Adler 1980). Toedter et al. (1988) concluded that "viewed as a whole, the literature on perinatal loss is largely unsystematic and based on psychiatric case studies or very small scale studies of mostly married middle-class couples" (p. 436).

Second-Trimester Spontaneous Abortion

Definition

Spontaneous abortion may be defined as the accidental loss of an embryo or fetus at any time between conception and 20 weeks of gestation (Hall et al. 1987). A second-trimester spontaneous abortion is usually considered to be one that occurs between 12 and 20 weeks (Hall et al. 1987; LaFerla 1986).

Incidence

It is estimated that approximately 15–20% of recognized pregnancies end in spontaneous abortion (LaFerla 1986), with more than 25% of these occurring after 15 weeks of gestation (Hall et al. 1987). The risk of aborting decreases with increasing lengths of gestation. It is lower in a subsequent pregnancy if the first abortus was karyotypically abnormal (Lauritsen 1976). The risk of second-trimester spontaneous abortion is relatively high in adolescence, decreases in the age range of 20–24 years, and gradually increases again after age 30 (LaFerla 1986).

Presentation

Spontaneous abortion in the second trimester, as in the first, can present in stages ranging from threatened to complete. *Threatened abortion* is diagnosed in an otherwise normal pregnancy when transcervical bleeding occurs before viability (LaFerla 1986). Threatened abortion occurs in 10–20% of pregnancies, approximately half of which end in abortion. The risk of later problems such as placenta previa and premature labor is higher after threatened abortion. With the possible exception of progesterone therapy for women with luteal phase defects, no interventions have been proven efficacious in preventing fetal wastage (Athanasiou et al. 1973).

An *inevitable abortion* is diagnosed when the cervix becomes effaced and dilated. It is usually accompanied by several days of bleeding and abdominal cramps. At times bleeding and cramping persist, despite conservative efforts to control them, without expulsion of the fetus. This condition is termed an *incomplete abortion* and is usually treated with dilatation and curettage early in the second trimester and with artificial induction of labor after about 14 weeks. A woman's consent to these procedures stresses her role in the decision to abort the fetus. *Complete abortion* is spontaneous expulsion of all of the products of conception. In some cases, the fetus will die for no obvious reason and without spontaneous contractions. This is termed a *missed abortion*. A brownish vaginal discharge may occur.

Abortions can recur because of several factors. If three or more spontaneous abortions occur in succession, the condition is termed *habitual abortion*. The risk of recurrence becomes increasingly higher with each successive abortion. For years habitual abortion was largely attributed to personality traits and other psychological factors. More recent literature suggests that the psychological problems identified in a woman who habitually aborts may be the result rather than the cause of frequent abortion. These problems may include difficulty in planning and anticipating, poor emotional control, an emphasis on conformity, strong feelings of dependency, a tendency to feel guilt, and neurosis (Seibel and Taymor 1982).

Psychological Response

The grief response after spontaneous abortion can be intense and is often accompanied by guilt—that is, "What did I do wrong?" (LaFerla 1986). A woman recovering from spontaneous abortion often lacks many of the supports of others who grieve (Rubin 1975). Hospitals are poorly organized for the care of a woman who aborts; she may not have told anyone she was pregnant, and she is unlikely to take part in rituals associated with mourning, such as having loved ones present at the time of loss or attending a funeral. In addition, she may refuse or be denied the opportunity to see her fetus, so she is left with fantasies about appearance, sex, and personality.

The literature on spontaneous abortion does not differentiate between first- and second-trimester experience in terms of psychological response, but some extrapolations can be made. Studies indicate that feelings of loss either remain the same or increase in intensity with gestational age (Hall et al. 1987; Toedter et al. 1988). Women who abort during the second trimester are more likely to have already worked through feelings of ambivalence about the pregnancy (Rubin 1975), to have felt the baby move, and to have told significant others about the pregnancy.

Pathological Grief Reaction

Numerous pathologic grief reactions to spontaneous abortion are described in the literature. They include nightmares about the abortion, abdominal pain and cramping similar to that which occurred during the abortion, headaches and backaches, vivid memories of the abortion events, frequent flashbacks to conversations or scenes from the date of the abortion, recurrent anniversary reactions on the date of the abortion or due date of birth, unwillingness to resume normal functions, persistent depression, intense focused anger, prolonged sadness and emotional lability when discussing the loss, a sensation of emotional flooding during stress or crisis, and clinging to symbols of the fetus (David 1975; Greene 1958; Kovacs and Beck 1978). Uncertainty, powerlessness, helplessness, guilt, shame, sadness, disbelief, frustration, anger, blame, recurrent disappointment, and substance abuse are symptoms of pathological grief resulting from spontaneous abortion. Feelings of guilt are often unrealistic, and they are most difficult for a woman and her partner to overcome (Hall et al. 1987). A woman generally has little warning of the abortion and therefore is unable to begin anticipatory preparation for the loss.

Possible predisposing factors for a pathological grief reaction after spontaneous abortion include a recent significant change in socioeconomic status, severe financial stress (Rubin 1975; Simon et al. 1969), the knowledge that the fetus was abnormal (Donnai and Harris 1981), previous loss of a child or parent (Kennell et al. 1970), and a history of depressive reactions. Other factors that may be associated with abnormal postabortion psychological states are a single and nulliparous status, ambivalent feelings about the pregnancy, cultural situations placing a higher premium on fertility, and previous emotional disorders (Rubin 1975; Simon et al. 1969). Psychotic reactions associated with spontaneous abortion occur most frequently after missed abortions because of the woman's difficulty with carrying a dead and defective fetus. Symptoms can range from psychotic agitation and turmoil to delusional denial and a search for second opinions. The woman may also attempt to abort the fetus herself (Hall et al. 1987).

Members of the medical profession have tended to ignore the psychological aspects of spontaneous abortion, possibly because of discomfort with grief, a feeling that grief is private, and a feeling that grief associated with spontaneous abortion is fairly minor compared with a loss later in the pregnancy or after the child is born. Spontaneous abortion is often associated with intense grief, however. It carries a risk of pathological sequelae (Hall et al. 1987), and it may not be related to gestational age (Peppers and Kna 1980).

Management

We recommend that, whenever possible, ultrasound studies be done to determine whether a fetus is alive, especially in cases of threatened second-trimester abortion. If a woman is hospitalized with continuing bleeding and the fetal heartbeat is detectable, we further recommend that this method of determining continuing life be provided to the woman on request.

Common methods of reassurance need to be reevaluated. For example, the tendency of many health professionals and laypersons is immediately to reassure a couple with the thought of future pregnancy or refer to the early age or probable abnormality of the fetus. These measures may intensify and prolong the grieving process by denying a woman permission to mourn and express her loss and by increasing her feelings of guilt.

Instead, specific attempts should be made by health care professionals to encourage and assist a woman and her family to work through the spontaneous abortion. Care should be taken to use appropriate terminology; for example, the word *abortion* should be replaced with *miscarriage* to avoid any connection with induced abortion. Psychotherapy and individual attention from the woman's physician have been shown to significantly reduce the incidence and severity of the grief response (Forrest et al. 1982) and should probably be provided at least to a limited extent (Bourne and Lewis 1984; Clyman et al. 1979; Parkes 1980; Raphael 1977). Everyone, including the woman's partner, involved in a spontaneous abortion should be encouraged to ask questions, accept his or her feelings, and express them with medical personnel and significant others. The family should be informed about the feelings that can be anticipated (Athanasiou et al. 1973).

Other specific topics that may be helpful to discuss include what happens to the fetal body, family expectations for the child, feelings and changes in self-concept, and difficulties the family may be having in planning. When appropriate, the family should be reassured that the loss was not their fault and that the outcome of the pregnancy would probably have been the same no matter what the woman had done. The effect on family members, including children, should be assessed and addressed, and potential sources of disagreement about the pregnancy (including its desirability) and the abortion should be discussed. The parents should be helped to think through how others could best support them. If the parents wish, friends and family members should be encouraged to acknowledge the loss by sending flowers, cards, and other expressions of sympathy.

If at any point a woman experiences symptoms of clinical depression or anxiety or becomes obsessionally preoccupied with the loss to the point of being dysfunctional, professional help should be advised (Bourne and Lewis 1984; Hall et al. 1987; LaFerla 1986). A routine postabortion follow-up appointment should always be made with the primary physician. At this time the patient should be reassessed for the symptoms of abnormal psychological response and referred promptly to a psychiatrist if such action is indicated. Group or individual psychotherapy may be helpful to explore such topics as fear of pregnancy and delivery, isolation and loneliness, relationships with friends and family, and the family's behavioral or genetic role in the loss (Athanasiou et al. 1973).

For a woman contemplating future pregnancy, particularly when more than one abortion has occurred, psychotherapy dealing with issues of loss, fear of pregnancy, effects on the family, and stress reduction may be helpful. This is an adjunct to a search for physiological causes (Seibel and Taymor 1982). Most abortions are caused by fetal abnormalities; if this is the case, most families can be reassured by the knowledge that abortions caused by this factor are less likely to recur. They may also be reassured as the pregnancy advances that the risk of abortion decreases with gestational age.

Second-Trimester Induced Abortion

Definition and Incidence

Second-trimester induced abortion is the artificial termination of pregnancy during the second trimester. More than 1.5 million abortions are performed in the United States each year (Olley 1985); this figure represents approximately one-third of this country's pregnancies (Henshaw et al. 1982). Only 9% of the 1980 U.S. abortions occurred after 12 weeks of gestation (Zakus and Wilday 1987), a decline of almost 2% during the previous 5 years. A similar decline is evident in all countries for which statistics are available (Tietze 1983). In 1981 in Canada, .2% of all legal abortions were performed after 20 weeks, compared to 1% in the United States. The incidence of second-trimester abortion is generally highest in those aged 0–17 years and gradually decreases to a low in those aged 30–34 years (Tietze 1983).

Many proposed and enacted recent laws address gestational age (or, more specifically, "viability") directly. These laws often impose unscientific or impracticable regulations for the determination of fetal ability to survive after delivery. These are probably related to the increased emotional weight of aborting a formed fetus and the desire to drive a popularly acceptable wedge into access to abortion in general. (Legal issues are covered in Chapter 4.)

Method

First-trimester abortions are often performed on an outpatient (Henshaw et al. 1982; Lewis et al. 1971) or day-care basis using menstrual regulation, vacuum aspiration, or dilatation and curettage techniques. Second-trimester abortions usually require hospitalization and are accomplished through dilatation and evacuation, stimulation of uterine contractions (hypertonic saline induction, prostaglandins), or major surgery (hysterotomy, hysterectomy) (Tietze 1983).

The complexity of the procedure—in terms of time, technical performance, cost, and medical risk—increases with the length of gestation, even within each trimester (Olley 1985). First-trimester abortion is a relatively simple procedure; second-trimester abortion "may involve several days in hospital (to allow for induction), a labor of three to eight hours, and the delivery of a recognizably human fetus" (Lewis et al. 1971, p. 607). Second-trimester abortion also carries a considerably higher risk of morbidity and mortality (Cates et al. 1977; Selik et al. 1981). Technical problems include a larger uterus and a larger fetus, requiring special instrumentation; an unripe cervix; and a changing amniotic fluid volume (Hern 1981). Saline and prostaglandin inductions carry higher risks of complication than dilatation and evacuation (Cates et al. 1977). They require more time, are more expensive, and are more painful than dilatation and evacuation. This is emotionally difficult for a woman (Rooks and Cates 1977).

Etiology

Those abortions performed in the second trimester are considered to be delayed. In a 1974 report in the United Kingdom, an average delay of 4 weeks was reported from the time a woman first contacted a physician to the time of abortion. In Canada in 1976, the average delay was 8 weeks (Olley 1985).

These delays can be system- or patient-induced. In one study, the health care system was found to be responsible for delays caused by misdiagnosis, late scheduling, and shortage of facilities in 26% of abortion patients (Mallory et al. 1972). In 1977, more than 500,000 women requesting an abortion in the United States were unable to obtain one (Forrest et al. 1982), and more than 50% of the second-trimester abortions reported in some areas (e.g., New York) were performed for nonresidents.

An abortion induced for medical reasons, such as fetal anomalies, may not be performed until the pregnancy reaches 18–24 weeks of gestation (Olley 1985). This type of abortion depends on the prior recognition of a high-risk pregnancy and the use of a technique that can detect the abnormality with a high degree of certainty. Such techniques generally are unreliable until after 16 weeks of gestation.

Studies indicate that reasons for patient delays include a failure to recognize the early signs of pregnancy, an inability to face the implications of pregnancy, a hesitancy in informing parents or physicians, and an initial decision to continue with the pregnancy (Henshaw et al. 1982). One study found a significant interaction among ego resilience, conflict and denial, and gestational age at the time of abortion, concluding that some delay may be needed to reach a high-quality decision, especially under conditions of conflict (Bracken and Kasl 1975). Psychotherapy may be particularly helpful in assisting women who are having difficulty to come to an earlier, well-considered decision.

Characteristics of Patients

The few studies directed at second-trimester abortion have primarily analyzed the demographic characteristics of women undergoing induced second-trimester abortion. Bracken and Kasl (1976) found that women undergoing second-trimester abortion in the United States were "significantly more likely than women undergoing first trimester abortion to be under 21 years old, single, have 0 or 1 living children, be black, have not completed high school, be Protestant, have been referred through clinic or university services, and to have not used a contraceptive at the time of conception" (p. 21). Johnstone and Vincent (1973) found a similar situation in Great Britain. Race and religion were not included in their list, but they found more women of lower social class, materially unsupported, or estranged from the putative father among women undergoing second-trimester abortions. Bracken and Kasl (1975) later advanced denial of pregnancy as another important characteristic. Kaltreider (1973), in a small descriptive study of postabortion women, found that for second-trimester aborters, the relationship with their parents was more often disturbed, their school and social histories suggested that they had been less successful, they had an increased sense of identity with their babies, they were more ambivalent regarding termination of the pregnancy, they were more interested in the resources available to help them to keep their children, they uniformly described a long period of denial that seemed to be an extension of a previous pattern of flight or of frenzied activity to avoid direct coping with uncomfortable situations, they had involved more people in the discussion, and several had presented themselves for abortion in response to peer pressure.

Psychological Responses

Although earlier studies on induced abortion suggested a high proportion of serious psychiatric illness after induced abortion, more recent reports have not confirmed this (Adler 1980; Olley 1985). Difficulties with methodology, such as lack of long-term follow-up activity, continue to hamper conclusions. Stresses include the undesired pregnancy and the reasons why it was conceived and is undesired, conflicts over the decision, the loss of the heir apparent, and violation of the body's integrity by the operation. A mild degree of emotional disturbance during the first 3 months after abortion is common, composed of a "transient reactive depression with nervousness and sleep disturbance" (Olley 1985, p. 181). Negative reactions are either responses to violating social, religious, and moral values (guilt, shame, and fear of disapproval) or responses to loss (regret, anxiety, depression, doubt, and anger). Single women and women who attend church frequently are more likely to exhibit society-based responses, those who find it difficult to make the abortion decision are more likely to exhibit internally based responses, and younger women tend to exhibit both types of response. Younger women tend to react more negatively than older women, unmarried women react more negatively than married women, and Roman Catholic women react more negatively than non-Catholics (Adler 1980).

Kaltreider (1973), in a descriptive study of a group of 18 women with similar backgrounds seeking abortion, found major differences in the response of first- and second-trimester aborters. Early aborters experienced a sense of relief and a desire to continue with life where they had left off; second-trimester aborters felt more mixed emotions, with a pattern of denial extending to the hospitalization. They reported a considerably more negative hospital experience than did first-trimester aborters. They often felt they had been inadequately prepared, found the experience uncomfortable, and had mixed emotions about the abortion procedure. Athanasiou et al. (1973), in a comparison of early and late aborters to women who delivered at term, concluded that there was little difference between the groups a year after abortion or delivery. In this study, three comparison groups were matched for demographic and socioeconomic variables from within the sample selected.

Predisposing Factors to Psychological Sequelae

Many of the predisposing factors associated with postabortion pathologic responses after induced abortion parallel the characteristics of spontaneous second-trimester aborters. Predisposing factors include a history of previous psychosocial instability, severe ambivalence, the significant involvement of outside pressure in the decision to abort, a decision made on medical grounds, and a history of poor interpersonal relationships (Olley 1985). Evidence suggests that the incidence and severity of negative response may be greater for a woman obtaining an abortion on medical grounds (Niswander and Patterson 1967; Peck and Marcus 1966; Simon et al. 1967). Such a woman is more likely to have a wanted pregnancy and is therefore more likely to experience a greater sense of loss (Adler 1980). Negative response may also be worse after fetal movement has been felt (Henshaw et al. 1982) or after saline induction, which results in 4–12 hours of active labor culminating in the delivery of a dead and recognizably human fetus (Adler 1980). Further research needs to be directed to second-trimester abortion to determine the risk of pathological sequelae and to identify optimal methods of treatment.

Treatment

Psychological assessment, support, and intervention should begin when a woman first presents herself for medical assistance with the pregnancy and should include postabortion screening for serious psychopathology and resolution of grief. Appropriate support and intervention beginning before the abortion may lead to an improvement in overall adjustment (Schmidt and Priest 1981). The goal should be to allay anxiety and assist the woman to the earliest decision possible by providing all necessary information and helping her to examine her feelings about her situation (Adler 1980); ensure that the woman is adequately prepared for the abortion procedure and the grieving process that is likely to follow (Athanasiou et al. 1973); and assist her with the resolution of negative feelings and prevent other postabortion problems, including those regarding future sexuality and parenthood (Bourne and Lewis 1984). The five steps of abortion decision making identified by Bracken and Kasl (1975) may be helpful. These are acknowledgment of pregnancy (Adler 1980), formulation of alternative outcomes (either delivery or abortion) (Athanasiou et al. 1973), selection of the outcome (Bourne and Lewis 1984), commitment to the chosen outcome (Bracken and Kasl 1986), and adherence to the decision (Bracken and Kasl 1975). Consideration should be given to reducing physical stress through choice of abortion techniques and provision of sensitive care. For those women undergoing procedures involving stimulation of labor, the presence of a support person should be encouraged and medication should be provided to limit discomfort. If negative sequelae develop, a decision should be made regarding the need for specialized counseling. The most appropriate intervention may be psychotherapy, although few studies have been done to assess its postabortion effectiveness. Group therapy may be best for some women, individual therapy for others (Adler 1980).

Conclusion

Approximately 25% of spontaneous abortions and 9% of therapeutic abortions occur during the second trimester. With the advent of more restrictive abortion laws and associated delays in obtaining an abortion, these numbers are expected to increase.

Recent studies suggest that the risks of serious or long-lasting sequelae are minimal after spontaneous or induced abortion; however, the results are not definitive, and few studies compare or differentiate between first- and second-trimester abortion concerns. Those that do differentiate between the trimesters have usually concentrated on the demographic and other characteristics of the aborter rather than on psychological outcome and treatment.

An analysis of these characteristics reveals that the second-trimester aborter may be more likely than the first-trimester aborter to experience post-abortion sequelae. Among other characteristics, the second-trimester aborter generally experiences a greater ambivalence toward abortion, receives more outside pressure to abort, has more psychosocial problems before the abortion, and is more likely to obtain an abortion on medical grounds. Each of these factors has been identified as a precursor to negative abortion sequelae.

Similar parallels are not evident in the spontaneous-abortion literature. Nevertheless, a woman who aborts spontaneously during the second trimester may also be at greater risk for postabortion sequelae because of such factors as increased procedural complexity, increased investment in the pregnancy, and recognition of fetal movement.

Further research is required to confirm and establish the significance of these relationships. Until such confirmation is available, any woman undergoing second-trimester abortion should probably receive careful pre-abortion and postabortion assessment and counseling from her primary physician. If signs of psychopathology become evident, the woman should be referred for psychiatric assessment and appropriate therapy.

References

Adler NE: Psychosocial issues of therapeutic abortion, in Psychosomatic Obstetrics and Gynecology. Edited by Youngs DD, Ehrhardt AA. New York, Appleton-Century-Crofts, 1980, pp 159–177

Athanasiou R, Oppel W, Michelson L, et al: Psychiatric sequelae to birth and induced early and late abortion: a longitudinal study. Fam Plann Perspect 5:227, 1973

Bourne S, Lewis E: Pregnancy after stillbirth or neonatal death: psychological risks and management. Lancet 2:31–33, 1984

Bracken MB, Kasl SV: Delay in seeking induced abortion. Am J Obstet Gynecol 121:1008–1019, 1975

Bracken MB, Kasl SV: Psychosocial correlates of delayed decisions to abort. Health Education Monographs 4:6–44, 1976

Bracken MB, Swigar ME: Factors associated with delay in seeking induced abortions. Am J Obstet Gynecol 114:10–12, 1972

Cates W Jr, Schulz KF, Grimes DA, et al: The effect of delay and method choice on the risk of abortion morbidity. Fam Plann Perspect 9:266, 1977

Clyman RF, Green C, Mikkelsen C, et al: Do patients utilize physician follow up after the death of their newborn? Pediatrics 64:665–667, 1979

David CJ: Grief mourning and pathological mourning. Prim Care 2:81–92, 1975

Donnai CN, Harris R: Attitudes of patients after "genetic" termination of pregnancy. Br Med J 282:621–622, 1981

Forrest GC, Standish E, Baum JD: Support after perinatal death: a study of support and counselling after perinatal bereavement. Br Med J 2:1475–1479, 1982

Greene A: Role of the vicarious object in the adaptation to object loss. Psychosom Med 20:344–350, 1958

Hall RCW, Beresford TP, Quinones JE: Grief following spontaneous abortion. Psychiatr Clin North Am 10:405–420, 1987

Henshaw SK, Forrest JD, Sullivan E, et al: Abortion services in the United States, 1979 and 1980. Fam Plann Perspect 14:5, 1982

Hern WM: Second-trimester abortion, in Abortion Practice. Philadelphia, PA, JB Lippincott, 1981, p 123–131

Johnstone FD, Vincent L: Factors affecting gestational age at termination of pregnancy. Lancet 2:717–719, 1973

Kaltreider NB: Emotional patterns related to delay in decision to seek legal abortion. Calif Med 118:23–27, 1973

Kennell JH, Slyter H, Klaus MH: The mourning response of parents to the death of a newborn infant. N Engl J Med 283:344–349, 1970

Kovacs M, Beck AT: Maladaptive cognitive structures and depression. Am J Psychiatry 13:525–537, 1978

LaFerla JJ: Spontaneous abortion. Clin Obstet Gynecol 13:105–114, 1986

Lauritsen JF: Aetiology of spontaneous abortion. Acta Obstet Gynecol Scand Suppl 52:1–29, 1976

Lewis SC, Lal S, Branch B, et al: Out-patient termination of pregnancy. Br Med J 4:606–610, 1971

Mallory GB, Rubenstein LZ, Drosness DL, et al: Factors responsible for delay in obtaining interruption of pregnancy. Obstet Gynecol 40:556–562, 1972

Niswander K, Patterson R: Psychological reaction to therapeutic abortion. Obstet Gynecol 19:702–706, 1967

Olley PC: Termination of pregnancy, in Psychological Disorders in Obstetrics and Gynaecology. Edited by Priest RG. London, Butterworth, 1985, pp 173–203

Parkes CM: Bereavement counselling: does it work? Br Med J 281:3–6, 1980

Peck A, Marcus H: Psychiatric sequelae of therapeutic interruption of pregnancy. J Nerv Ment Dis 143:417–425, 1966

Peppers LG, Kna RJ: Maternal reactions to involuntary fetal/infant death. Psychiatry 43:156–159, 1980

Raphael B: Preventive intervention with the recently bereaved. Arch Gen Psychiatry 34:1450–1454, 1977

Rooks JB, Cates W: Emotional impact of D&E vs instillation. Fam Plann Perspect 9:276–277, 1977

Rubin R: Maternal tasks in pregnancy. MCN 4:143–153, 1975

Schmidt R, Priest RG: The effects of termination of pregnancy: a follow-up study of psychiatric referrals. Br J Med Psychol 54:267–276, 1981

Seibel MM, Taymor ML: Emotional aspects of infertility. Fertil Steril 37:137–145, 1982

Selik RM, Cates W Jr, Tyler CW Jr: Behavioral factors contributing to abortion deaths: a new approach to mortality studies. Obstet Gynecol 58:631, 1981

Simon N, Senturia A, Rothman D: Psychiatric illness following therapeutic abortion. Am J Psychiatry 124:97–103, 1967

Simon NM, Rothman D, Goff JT, et al: Psychological factors related to spontaneous and therapeutic abortion. Am J Obstet Gynecol 104:799–808, 1969

Tietze C: Induced Abortion: A World Review. New York, Population Council, 1983

Toedter LJ, Lasker JN, Alhadeff JM: The perinatal grief scale: development and initial validation. Am J Orthopsychiatry 58:435–449, 1988

Zakus G, Wilday S: Adolescent abortion option. Soc Work Health Care 12:77–91, 1987

Chapter 12

Racial and Ethnic Influences: The Black Woman and Abortion

Irma J. Bland, M.D.

The difference in attitude among women about the issue of abortion may be individual and idiosyncratic, dependent on particular sociodemographic variables, or it may be the result of racial or ethnic influences. In this chapter, I make no attempt to cover all racial and ethnic groups, but I focus on one particular group and, where appropriate, attempt to elucidate the potential influence of these issues in general.

There are tremendous intraethnic and cultural variations among members of any ethnic group as a result of income, occupation, area of origin, religion, age, sex, and education (Harwood 1981). Regardless of ethnic origin, the more alike people are, particularly in educational status and socioeconomic class, the more their ideas, perceptions, attitudes, and beliefs may converge. Yet members of an ethnic group still retain their ethnic beliefs and are likely to resort to them under particular circumstances— for example, when stressed or faced with illness. The issue of abortion falls within such a category in which racial and ethnic influences may potentially play a significant role.

The history of blacks in America lends itself to this task and offers some interesting insights. During times of slavery, blacks were separated from their families and usually were not permitted to formally sanction their unions through marriage (Ladner 1972). All children born were theoretically illegitimate, yet they were accepted into the family, an old tradition that remains within the ethnic culture of the black community. What are the enduring psychological effects of history on black women's perceptions of and attitudes about pregnancy, motherhood, and the termination of pregnancy by abortion? Ethnic issues may influence not only access to abortion but also attitudes, perceptions, the process of decision making, the nature of psychological conflicts engendered, and the course of psychological adaptation after abortion.

We live in a heterogeneous, multicultural society, yet true cultural pluralism psychologically has not been achieved. The premise of a dominant culture causes the tendency to dichotomize life as good or bad, superior or inferior, and right or wrong (Bell et al. 1983). Disregard for the internal and external frames of reference of different ethnic groups perpetuates faulty treatment alliances and interventions, and it ultimately impedes effective delivery of health care. These issues may play a significant role in the perception of abortion as an option (or not an option) for women of different ethnic groups (Crossley et al. 1977; Darity and Turner 1972; Schwartz and Abramowitz 1975) and in the way in which individuals from different racial and ethnic groups are dealt with by health care providers. Health care providers must remain objective yet aware of the particular racial and ethnic value-laden issues that must be confronted and worked through. This is essential for health care providers to assist women of different ethnic groups to choose freely and to come to a decision about an unwanted pregnancy based on real needs, circumstances, and psychological realities and to be better able, when necessary, to facilitate their postabortion adaptation.

Historical Background

The continuing psychological influence of an ethnic group's history should not be underestimated. Remnants of that history are passed down from generation to generation and continue to influence perspective, attitudes, and behavior. As with individuals, the nature of one's fears, conflicts, defenses, and modes of adaptation are all shaped by early childhood traumas and relationships. So too there is a cultural transmission within groups intergenerationally. The case is telling for blacks, who, because of the color of their skin, remain forever subject to symbolic reminders of their history through racial discrimination, hatred, negative projection, and stereotyping. They are denied opportunities for their dreams to be realized, and subsequently there is a socioeconomic blight for the masses of the group. Thus, no matter how many centuries have passed, no matter how far some blacks have progressed beyond their history, there remains embedded in the fabric of American society reminders that reverberate in the psyches of black people—the history of their beginnings in America as slaves and all of that history's ramifications. This reminder maintains and perpetuates from generation to generation old attitudes, fears, perceptions, and defensive operations.

The ancestry of black people lies in Africa, a land of heritage and tradition, of strong tribal kinship and extended family ties. In contrast, as slaves in America, blacks became strangers in an alien culture, uprooted from family, friends, and culture, and were not allowed to assimilate the new culture. To avoid rebellion, members of a tribe were separated and formal marriage between slaves was usually forbidden (Bernard 1966; Franklin 1980; Pinkey 1987; Tardy et al. 1976). Thus all children born during slavery were in essence born out of wedlock or illegitimate. Yet these children were accepted into the family, not penalized or held responsible for their parents' situations, an old tradition that still lives within the black community.

Motherhood for the black woman descended from the African mother whose maternal attitude for her child was shaped and fixed before it was born by various tribal customs and taboos. Rodgers-Rose (1980) described how, from the moment of conception, the African woman was expected to give her complete attention to the needs and desires of her child. Men were not allowed to interfere. When she was pregnant, the woman was expected to leave the house of her husband and return to the house of her father until the baby was born. She would return to the house of her husband when the child was about 3 years old and properly weaned. She was not to allow herself to run the risk of conceiving another child before then.

The African mother's love for her children has been described as "neither suppressed by the restraints, nor diverted by the solicitudes of civilized life and is everywhere conspicuous" (Frazier 1966, p. 33). Yet the black woman in slavery met challenges that undoubtedly created conflict with this maternal heritage:

> To pregnant women who formed a part of the slave caravans motherhood meant only a burden and an accentuation of their miseries. Maternal feeling was choked and dried up in mothers who had to bear children, in addition to loads of corn or rice on their back during marches of eight to fourteen hours. Nor did life in the slave pens on the coast, where they were chained and branded and sometimes starved, mitigate the sufferings of motherhood. (Frazier 1966, pp. 34–35)

During slavery, black women were made concubines for their slave masters, and both black women and men were used as breeders. Often slave women gave birth to a succession of "unwanted" children. Although some women were shattered by the experiences, many also survived. It required heroic efforts for a black slave woman to maintain the bonds and to avoid the destruction of her maternal feelings for her unwanted child. At the same time, slave women had to surrender and endure forced separation as they witnessed the selling of their own "wanted" children and were paralyzed with grief. Yet they were still required to nurture and suckle the children of their slave masters (Frazier 1966).

Pregnancy and motherhood for black women in slavery was an ambivalent enterprise at best. In contrast to the heritage of her African forebears, the black slave woman was denied the traditional customs and rituals attendant to her role as mother. During slavery, she was defined in terms of her breeding capacity, and she had no opportunity to properly plan or to space her children. When they were born, she was immediately separated from them to return to the fields and had to leave them in the care of older siblings or elderly women. She worked, suffered, and struggled, taking responsibility and caring for her children after work hours. Yet she lived in constant fear of their being taken away. Slavery may have transformed the structure of the mother-child relationship from that of its African heritage, but it did not destroy that bond. On the contrary, through this suffering, adversity, ambivalence, and conflict it is likely to have made it grow even stronger (Rodgers-Rose 1980).

Access, Availability, and Use of Abortion

Women have obtained access to and used abortion as a means of terminating undesired pregnancies since time immemorial, with and without the legal sanction to do so. When the U.S. Supreme Court legalized abortion in the *Roe v. Wade* (1973) decision, women's choices were more open to public scrutiny and scientific research. Various studies and surveys have examined women's attitudes about abortion (Granberg and Granberg 1980; Jones and Westoff 1978), characteristics of women who approve and disapprove of abortion (Henshaw 1987; Henshaw and O'Reilly 1983; Henshaw and Silverman 1988), and the rates of abortion use (Tietze 1983).

In the years preceding the legalization of abortion, we began to see an increasing liberalization of attitudes. By mid-1982 abortion was allowed in the United States pretty much on demand. It was possible for a woman to obtain an abortion within the first trimester on broad social grounds— for example, the unmarried status of the mother or financial problems. Although the likelihood of a woman getting an abortion may differ across cultural groups, women's reasons for seeking abortion are similar and fall into three categories: 1) nonoptimal mating (unmarried status, ambiguous paternity, rape, and incest); 2) health (threat to mother's health and deformity of fetus); and 3) social welfare (finances and family size) (Shain 1986; Torres and Forrest 1988).

Did the legalization of abortion, however, mean ready availability or access for all women? Perhaps not, and especially not for women of lower socioeconomic and educational status or for those who were geographically located outside major metropolitan areas, where these services were accessible. This was true across groups and was less a function of racial and ethnic variables per se. On the other hand, differential use (as compared to access and availability) is more likely to be influenced by racial and ethnic variables. Use would be determined by decision and choice if access and availability were constant across racial and ethnic groups. What would influence that choice is likely to be determined by an individual's cultural values and beliefs.

In examining the intermediate determinants of racial differences in the 1980 U.S. nonmarital fertility rates, Cutright and Smith (1988) demonstrated that a major contributor was lower abortion ratios (the number of abortions per 1,000 live births) for unmarried black women (across age groups) than for unmarried white women. As Cutright and Smith suggested, this is likely to be as much (if not more) a reflection of ethnic and cultural acceptance of the birth of the child to the unmarried woman as it is a reflection of access or availability of abortion services, to the extent that differential use reflects decision and choice and not access and availability. This seems to imply that a black woman's use of abortion as a means to terminate an unplanned or unintended pregnancy is influenced by the ethnic and cultural values of blacks.

The characteristic profile of the woman who chooses abortion has generally been cited as predominantly young, white, unmarried, and with a metropolitan residence. She is likely to have had few previous births and some college education. She decides to have an abortion because of an unplanned, unintended pregnancy. She faces either physical risks or significant pressure against a nonmarital birth and refuses childbearing, which would mean forgoing social and economic opportunities (Henshaw 1987; Henshaw and O'Reilly 1983; Powell-Griner and Trent 1987). In Shain's (1986) analysis, the woman is also likely to be younger than 49 years and not strongly committed to organized religion (especially Roman Catholicism or Fundamentalism). She has liberal rather than conservative traditional attitudes regarding women's roles in life, premarital sex, sex education, and civil liberties.

Abortion Attitudes and Perceptions: A Survey of Black Women

Few systematic efforts have been made to look specifically at different subgroups of women (e.g., black women or subsections of that group) regarding attitudes and perceptions about abortion. How do black women differ, and how are they similar to other groups of women regarding the issue of abortion? What are the unique issues within this group, and what can we understand from black women about the racial and ethnic influences in abortion? Which factors converge with other ethnic groups as members move into similar educational and socioeconomic ranks, and which influences remain unaltered?

To examine these issues, an expanded clinical study was conducted with a volunteer study group. The participants were given an open-ended questionnaire in a structured interview exploring abortion in regard to the continuity of their life experiences as black women. Interviews were recorded on audiotape to ensure accuracy and to analyze the data.

Sociodemographic Analysis

The 50 women who composed this study group ranged in age from 15 to 86 years. The largest group (62%) fell within the main childbearing years, 25–44 years old (see Table 1). Approximately two-thirds (68%) of the women were unmarried: 50% were single or had never married, and 18% were separated, divorced, or widowed. Nearly 50% of the women had no children. As shown in Table 2, most (84%) of these women reported that they considered abortion an option to terminate an unwanted pregnancy: 18% had had abortions, 12% had considered having an abortion, and 54% would consider having an abortion. Only 16% said that they would never consider abortion. The women in this study were predominantly Protestant, with 62% non-Catholic and 38% Catholic. This was a relatively educated, working, career-bound group of women. Approximately one-third of them were professionals or held business administrative positions. About one-fourth were students, ranging from high school to graduate school. Only 4% were housewives.

The Fate of an Unwanted Pregnancy

What is the likelihood that an unplanned, unwanted pregnancy will end in abortion? It depends on a woman's definition of an unwanted pregnancy and the ethnic-laden value associated with that definition. When asked for the primary circumstance in which abortion would be considered, each of these women had her own idea of what constituted an unwanted pregnancy and what ranked as the most important circumstance in which to consider abortion (see Table 3).

Not unexpectedly, as many women defined an unwanted pregnancy as one that resulted from forced conception (32%) as considered it the primary circumstance in which they would consider abortion (32%). Forced conception might be considered the least ethnic value-laden circumstance that these women used to define an unwanted pregnancy. On the other hand, although 26% of these women defined an unwanted pregnancy as one that interrupted life goals, none of the sample (0%) cited that particular circumstance as a primary consideration for abortion. Similarly, a much larger percentage of women defined an unwanted pregnancy as one that created

Table 1.   Sociodemographic analysis of study participants

	n	%
Age (years)		
15–19	7	14
20–24	6	12
25–34	10	20
35–44	21	42
45–54	3	6
≥55	3	6
Marital status		
Single	25	50
Separated/divorced/widowed	9	18
Married	16	32
Religion		
Catholic	19	38
Baptist	24	48
Other Protestant[a]	7	14
Education[b]		
Grade school	4	8
High school	21	42
College graduate	12	24
Graduate degree	13	26
Occupation		
Housewife	2	4
Student	13	26
Clerical/sales/technician	10	20
Semiskilled worker	8	16
Business/administrative	6	12
Professional	11	22
Number of children		
None	24	48
1–2	15	30
3–4	8	16
≥5	3	6

[a] Includes Lutheran (3), Methodist (3), and Spiritualist (1).
[b] Education completed.

an economic hardship (24%) than would actually consider this a reason for an abortion (6%). Despite the anticipated hardship, there was a self-sacrificing attitude, and many women felt responsibility to the unborn child, no matter how hard the task.

Although few women in this group defined an unwanted pregnancy as one out of wedlock (6%), nearly four times as many (22%) would consider this circumstance when considering abortion. Similarly, although only 2% could conceive of a health risk making a pregnancy unwanted, 16% would consider a health risk a reason to consider abortion. Twelve percent of the group indicated that there would be no circumstance in which abortion should be a consideration.

Table 2.   Attitudes about abortion

	n	%
Position on abortion		
For	33	66
Extraordinary circumstances only[a]	5	10
Against	12	24
Attitude change in past 10 years		
Change	16	32
No change	34	68
Attitude has become[b]		
More liberal	13	81
More conservative	3	19
Factor most influencing attitude		
Family upbringing	8	16
Religion	9	18
Social issues	26	52
Experience with abortion	6	12
Unknown	1	2
Abortion is a form of genocide		
Yes	9	18
No	41	82
Use of abortion		
Have had	9	18
Considered having	6	12
Would consider having	15	30
Would consider in extraordinary circumstances only	12	24
Would never consider	8	16
Position on adoption as alternative solution		
Would consider	6	12
Against adoption	44	88

[a] Extraordinary circumstances would include rape, incest, threat to mother's life, or fetus known to be defective.
[b] Only that proportion whose attitudes changed ($n = 16$).

Attitudes About Abortion

The attitudes and perceptions about abortion varied widely among this group of women (see Table 2). There were interesting variations within families, between mothers and daughters, between sisters, and between best friends. Each woman had her own individual, very personal, at times idiosyncratic ideas about the subject. Each had seriously struggled with the issue and had an understanding of those factors most influential in shaping her attitudes.

Most of the women (76%) were supportive of abortion, 10% of whom qualified their position as supporting abortion under "extraordinary circumstances only." Twenty-four percent were opposed to abortion, but when asked to cite the circumstances in which they would consider abor-

Table 3. Comparison of definition of unwanted pregnancy and circumstances to consider abortion

	Definition of unwanted pregnancy		Circumstance to consider abortion	
	n	%	n	%
Forced conception[a]	16	32	16	32
Health risk to mother/child	1	2	8	16
Interrupts life goals	13	26		
Out of wedlock/unstable relationship	3	6	11	22
Economic hardship	12	24	3	6
Emotional hardship	4	8	5	10
Want no (no more) children			1	2
No circumstance			6	12
Could not define	1	2		

[a] Forced conception indicated a pregnancy that resulted from rape or incest.

tion, 12% of this group fell out, leaving only 12% standing firm in their position against abortion ("under no circumstance"). All of these women, both for and against abortion, struggled with the issue of morality. Some successfully found a point of reconciliation with the moral issue, whereas others seemed to suspend morality as needed when confronted with real-life situations.

Most of these women had held constant in their position on abortion for the past 10 years (68%). For those whose attitude had changed (32%), a few had become more conservative with maturation (19%). An overwhelming majority, however, had become more liberal (81%), citing social issues as influential in that regard. Social issues stood out as the most important factor influencing a position on abortion for most of the women in this group (52%), much more important than family upbringing (16%) or religion (18%). Social issues referred to the increasing feminization of poverty, child abuse, and adolescent pregnancy. There was no correlation of statistical significance between a position on abortion and age, marital status, or occupation. Correlations that approached significance ($P < .10$) were between a position on abortion and religion ($r = -.26$, $P = .06$) and between a position on abortion and education completed ($r = .26$, $P = .07$). Proabortion women tended to be non-Catholic and had higher levels of education completed. An even higher correlation ($P < .01$) was seen between a position on abortion and the most influential factor determining that position. Abortion support showed a negative correlation with religion ($r = -.55$, $P = .0001$) and a positive correlation with social issues ($r = .53$, $P = .0001$).

Religious orientation, which can be strongly bound to culture, plays a significant role in attitudes about, perceptions of, and positions on abortion.

All of the women struggled with the issue of morality in the context of their religious upbringing and current religious affiliations. There was a striking difference between religious teachings on abortion among Catholics and non-Catholics. Most Catholics indicated that their church was vocal and overtly opposed to abortion and identified it as immoral. Non-Catholics, however, did not consider abortion an issue within their church, or they considered it one for which no vocal position was taken by the church. It was much easier for the non-Catholics of this group to reconcile themselves as being proabortion. Yet even the non-Catholics maintained that prayer or religious counseling is an important aspect of their decision making and anticipated postabortion adaptation (see Table 4). With increasing education, ideas bound to religion tended to be somewhat less influential.

The results of the analysis of the responses from the women of this group are consistent with previous observations. As delineated by Shain (1986), sociodemographic variables appear to have less impact in explaining overall attitudes about and positions on abortion. Stronger predictors appear to be the importance of religion (Legge 1983), the level of education (except for Catholics, for whom their deeply entrenched Catholicism more often supersedes education), and perhaps racial and ethnic value-laden issues.

Racial and Ethnic Value-Laden Issues

Genocide

Among those issues considered racial or ethnic value-laden within the black community is genocide. How important is the fear and perception of genocide on black women in their sense of free choice regarding abortion? When asked, "Do you consider abortion to be a form of genocide?" the overwhelming majority of the participants (82%) said no, whereas 18% said yes. A high correlation was seen between abortion as a form of genocide and a position on abortion ($r = -.50$, $P = .0002$), religion as the most influential determinant ($r = .42$, $P = .0026$), and level of education ($r = .25$, $P = .08$). Those who perceived abortion to be a form of genocide tended to be more influenced by religion, less educated, and against abortion. A review of contemporary and historical materials by Darity and Turner (1972) raised questions in earlier years about the fear of genocide and showed an inverse relationship between use of family-planning methods and genocidal convictions.

Adoption

Historically, from clinical impression and borne out by empirical data, black women are overwhelmingly against adoption as an alternative res-

Table 4.   Psychological issues, resolutions, and postabortion adaptation

	n	%
Issue most associated with decision to terminate unwanted pregnancy		
Guilt/moral issues	33	66
Shame	2	4
Sense of loss	7	14
None	8	16
Resolution		
Work through alone/adjust in time	5	10
Support of family/friends	8	16
Professional counseling	9	18
Prayer/religious counseling	20	40
No answer	8	16
Issue most associated with decision not to terminate unwanted pregnancy		
Acceptance of/bonding with child	15	30
Single parenthood	9	18
Interruption of personal/career goals	3	6
Emotional hardship	14	28
Economic hardship	9	18
Resolution		
Work through alone/adjust in time	25	50
Support of family/friends	13	26
Professional counseling	2	4
Prayer/religious counseling	8	16
No answer	2	4
Anticipate emotional problems after abortion		
Yes	35	70
No	15	30
Duration of postabortion problems		
Acute only	4	8
Long term	32	64
None	14	28
Nature of postabortion problems		
Sense of loss	11	22
Guilt	25	50
None	14	28
Need for professional help		
Yes	26	52
No	10	20
No answer	14	28

olution to an unwanted pregnancy (see Table 2). Eighty-eight percent of these women reported that they were against adoption. Abortion was a more ethnically permissible and thus psychologically acceptable alternative to resolve an unwanted pregnancy. Otherwise, these women would keep a baby before giving it up for adoption, regardless of the circumstances.

Adoption was not a culturally permissible option or alternative solution to an unwanted pregnancy.

A positive correlation was seen between a position on adoption and age ($r = .30$, $P = .04$), education ($r = .30$, $P = .03$), and occupation ($r = .38$, $P = .0065$). Older and better-educated women with higher occupational status tended to be against adoption. Although these women were in a better position to keep their babies, more was at issue here. Interestingly, the younger women (younger than 20 years), a new generation, had been socialized to adoption as a solution to unintended pregnancy, perhaps in association with the epidemic of adolescent pregnancy. They considered adoption an even higher-ranked option than abortion.

Psychological Issues, Resolutions, and Postabortion Adaptation

The decision to terminate an unwanted pregnancy for the majority of these women (66%) was most associated with guilt or moral issues instead of a sense of loss (14%). Whether for or against abortion, the issue of morality and guilt, the idea of taking a life, was anticipated to be a major psychological issue (see Table 4). Sixteen percent anticipated no major problems. More often than not, these women indicated that they would turn to others for help. Prayer or religious counseling was considered most important for 40%, whereas 18% would seek professional counseling and 16% would seek support from family and friends. Only 10% expected that they could work through this alone or "adjust in time."

Regarding the decision not to terminate an unwanted pregnancy, 30% of the group expected the most significant problem to be accepting and bonding with the child and 28% expected the most significant problem to be emotional hardship. Only 6% considered interruption of personal or career goals most significant. The means of resolution in this context were somewhat different from what they were with a decision to terminate. Under this circumstance (a decision not to terminate), 50% of this group expected to work through this alone or adjust in time.

A majority of these women (70%) anticipated emotional problems after abortion. Unanimously they anticipated depression; 50% expected it to be the result of guilt, whereas 22% expected it to be associated with a sense of loss. The majority of these women expected long-term problems for more than a year (64%), and more than 50% anticipated the need for professional help in their postabortion adaptation.

Summary and Discussion

The more women of different racial and ethnic groups converge regarding their economic and educational attainment, life perspective, and goals (i.e., the more acculturated to the middle class), the more alike they become regarding their choices about abortion. This indeed may be true in regard to the final outcome. Yet what the women in this study demonstrated is that the path to reach that outcome psychologically may be very different, as influenced by the history of the racial or ethnic group and the particular ethnic value-laden issues that must be internally worked through and reconciled.

This was an expanded clinical study that used a volunteer, racially homogeneous group of women. Although by no means exhaustive or representative of all black women, the study of this subgroup was illustrative of the interplay and potential impact of racial and ethnic influences and abortion. What these women demonstrated is that a decision about abortion is an individual one, and there is tremendous variation in women's attitudes and perceptions. Regardless of one's final position (for or against), there is an active, internal struggle to reconcile remnants of family upbringing, historically and culturally binding issues of a particular racial or ethnic group, and self-oriented aspirations.

The fate of a pregnancy that is poorly timed or that occurs under unfavorable circumstances first depends on a woman's definition of an unwanted pregnancy and the freedom she feels in exercising options that are available to her. Racial and ethnic issues may significantly influence a woman's concept of an unwanted pregnancy and dictate the options that are culturally permissible to resolve it.

In most women's lives there is a substantial overlap in their perceptions of unwanted pregnancies interrupting life goals and producing economic hardship. Even though the women in this group could conceive of these circumstances as defining an unwanted pregnancy, racial and ethnic value-laden influences dictated their choices. Regardless of circumstances of birth, potential interruption of life goals, or economic hardship, the women felt a responsibility to the unborn child, which superseded personal comfort or self-oriented goals. Even if they risked allowing self-oriented needs and desires to take precedence, this remained an issue that had to be worked through and resolved psychologically for them.

Sociodemographic variables have only a limited role in determining a woman's attitudes and perceptions about abortion. Religion and education are much stronger determinants. Increased levels of education appeared to allow broader perspectives, diminishing to some extent restrictions of choice as a result of racial or ethnic influences. Similarly, increased education diminished culturally bound religious restrictions, except in regard to Catholicism. Despite freer exercise of choice, these again remained issues of significant conflict, which in the aftermath had to be worked through and reconciled.

Certain issues may be identified that are of special importance (in particular, racial and ethnic groups) and that directly influence or indirectly interface with abortion. In the past, genocide was considered a particular fear of blacks in regard to family planning in general and abortion in particular. The women who did associate abortion with genocide were overwhelmingly against abortion. Although a less acute or pervasive issue in the 1990s, it is a remnant influenced by race and ethnicity within certain subgroups of blacks, a remnant that one must be aware of and sensitive to.

Historically, black women have been less likely to adopt out their babies. Even though babies may be turned over to a grandmother or other relative, formal adoption has not been culturally sanctioned. Most of these women were emphatically against adoption as a solution for an unwanted pregnancy. There was more of a retention of this ethnic belief in older women uninfluenced by increased education, occupation, or level of sophistication.

Whatever the final outcome regarding the fate of an unwanted pregnancy, regardless of the position a woman ultimately takes, there remains a need to work through conflicts and reach points of reconciliation with racial and ethnic issues of the group. Most of these women anticipated the need for professional help after abortion, yet they still retained their culture-bound religious orientation and saw prayer and religious counseling as significant factors in their resolution attempts. This was, however, adjunctive to professional counseling rather than a substitute for it.

Roe v. Wade (1973) essentially granted the fundamental constitutional right to women in general to terminate unwanted pregnancy. For black women in particular it ultimately allowed freer access to abortion and psychologically granted a sense of permission to accept one's personal goals and self needs as legitimate and a sense of empowerment to control the destiny of their lives and the lives of their unborn children. The U.S. Supreme Court's *Webster v. Reproductive Health Services* (1989) decision conveys the assumption that abortion is no longer a fundamental right of women. It gives the states the right to impose new restrictions and places restrictions on use of public services for abortion. It is likely that this decision will ultimately undermine this newly found sense of empowerment, widening the gap between black women and further encumbering the psychological work and resolution of racial and ethnic conflicts.

It is essential that the dynamic interface of racial and ethnic influences be appreciated, understood, and addressed. Only then can we most effectively facilitate the working through of issues that women of different racial and ethnic groups must confront when faced with an unwanted pregnancy and the possibility of abortion—regardless of the final decision.

References

Bell C, Bland IJ, Houston E, et al: Enhancement of knowledge and skills for psychiatric treatment of black populations, in Mental Health and People of Color.

Edited by Chunn JC, Dunston PJ, Ross-Sheriff F. Washington, DC, Howard University Press, 1983, pp 205–237

Bernard J: Marriage and Family Among Negroes. Englewood Cliffs, NJ, Prentice-Hall, 1966

Crossley B, Abramowitz SI, Weitz LJ: Race and abortion: disconfirmation of the genocide hypothesis in a clinical analogue. Int J Psychiatry Med 8:35–42, 1977

Cutright P, Smith H: Intermediate determinants of racial differences in 1980 U.S. nonmarital fertility rates. Fam Plann Perspect 20:119–123, 1988

Darity WA, Turner CB: Family planning, race, consciousness and the fear of race genocide. Am J Public Health 62:1454–1459, 1972

Franklin JH: From Slavery to Freedom: A History of Negro Americans, 5th Edition. New York, Knopf, 1980

Frazier EF: Motherhood in bondage, in The Negro Family in the United States, 2nd Edition. Chicago, IL, University of Chicago Press, 1966, pp 33–49

Granberg D, Granberg BW: Abortion attitudes, 1965–1980 trends and determinants. Fam Plann Perspect 12:250–261, 1980

Harwood H (ed): Ethnicity and Medical Care. Cambridge, MA, Harvard University Press, 1981

Henshaw SK: Characteristics of U.S. women having abortions 1982–1983. Fam Plann Perspect 19:5–9, 1987

Henshaw SK, O'Reilly K: Characteristics of abortion patients in the United States, 1979 and 1980. Fam Plann Perspect 15:5–16, 1983

Henshaw SK, Silverman J: The characteristics and prior contraceptive use of U.S. abortion patients. Fam Plann Perspect 20:158–168, 1988

Jones E, Westoff C: How attitudes toward abortion are changing. Journal of Population 1:5–21, 1978

Ladner JA: Tomorrow's Tomorrow: The Black Woman. New York, Doubleday, 1972

Legge JS: The determinants of attitudes toward abortion in the American electorate. Western Political Quarterly 36:479–490, 1983

Pinkey A: Black Americans, 3rd Edition. Englewood Cliffs, NJ, Prentice-Hall, 1987

Powell-Griner E, Trent K: Sociodemographic determinants of abortion in the U.S. Demography 24:553–561, 1987

Rodgers-Rose L (ed): The Black Woman. Beverly Hills, CA, Sage, 1980

Roe v. Wade, 410 U.S. 113 (1973)

Schwartz JM, Abramowitz SI: Value related effects on psychiatric judgement. Arch Gen Psychiatry 32:1525–1532, 1975

Shain RN: A cross cultural history of abortion. Clin Obstet Gynecol 13:1–17, 1986

Tardy WJ, Lightfoot OB, Spiro HR, et al: Cultural Issues in Contemporary Psychiatry: The Inner City Black. Philadelphia, PA, SK&F, 1976

Tietze C: Induced Abortion: A World Review, 5th Edition. New York, Population Council, 1983

Torres A, Forrest JD: Why do women have abortions. Fam Plann Perspect 20:169–176, 1988

Webster v. Reproductive Health Services, 109 S.Ct. 3040 (1989)

Chapter 13

Adolescents and Abortion

Judith H. Gold, M.D., F.R.C.P.(C)

Jane, age 30, asked her therapist to see her 14-year-old daughter, Mary. Mary's long-standing problems with schoolwork and peer interactions were growing more troublesome to both of them and had increased somewhat since her therapeutic abortion 1 month previously. She was in the eighth grade in a junior high school that served a mainly upper-middle-class neighborhood, but her friends were school dropouts or academic underachievers. Mary felt that the teachers singled her out unfairly and that her classmates looked down on her.

Jane had become pregnant at age 15 and had raised Mary herself but with financial assistance from the father. Mary spent holidays with her father (also age 30) and his second wife and children. The father rarely remembered birthdays or holidays without a reminder from Jane, and Mary had many rushes of ambivalent feelings toward him. Jane was a university student whose studies were frequently interrupted by exacerbations of a chronic neurological illness that had only recently been definitely diagnosed. She was often bedridden or fatigued and would then require assistance from Mary.

Mary dressed appropriately for her age, but her conversation was sprinkled with comments obviously copied from her mother in an attempt to sound more mature. She had been moved from school to school as her mother changed jobs, was ill, or returned to the university over the years. Thus her peer relationships had been transient and she was accustomed to her mother's friends. Mary had attended her junior high school for 2 years and finally had some friends. They formed a small group on the fringe of the school population—socially, academically, and physically.

Mary and her friends started to smoke cigarettes about a year before, and they used alcohol regularly. They were not interested in street drugs, mainly because the other children were using them. They dressed differently from their school peers and resisted schoolwork. The girls were very competitive among themselves for the boys in the crowd and alternated best friends. They spent hours talking to each other on the telephone and looked to each other when in need of refuge from the troubled homes in which they all lived.

Mary began spending all of her time after school with 16-year-old Peter, who was unemployed, having left school the previous year. He lived with his alcoholic and abusive father and soon was demanding her constant attention and affection. Mary enjoyed being needed by him and the status with her friends that came from having a steady boyfriend. She also liked the cuddling and holding. Mary had reached menarche at age 12; her menstrual periods were irregular. The need for contraception had never occurred to her, even though Peter urged her to have sexual intercourse. She eventually consented to make him happy and to appease her own curiosity. She became pregnant immediately but did not recognize the cause of her morning nausea. Jane took her to the family physician, and the diagnosis was made. Mother and daughter agreed immediately that Mary must have an abortion. Mary stated clearly that she was a child and was totally unprepared emotionally to sustain a pregnancy. Furthermore, she did not want to repeat the struggles her mother had had in raising her.

Mary's pregnancy was terminated at 6 weeks of gestation. She did not tell her friends or her boyfriend; however, she determined to stop seeing Peter because she was certain he would want to have intercourse again. She was greatly relieved by this decision and said she would need to be "more mature emotionally" before she became sexually involved again. Now Mary began to worry about her poor school performance. Jane became concerned about her lack of parental control and guidance. In trying to establish a new role with Mary, Jane asked her therapist for assistance by referring her daughter for treatment.

This clinical vignette illustrates many of the features associated with teenage pregnancy. Adolescence is the voyage from child to adult. Epidemiological research has demonstrated that most people sail through adolescence with minor difficulties, but the remainder often cause themselves and others much anger and unhappiness (Offer and Offer 1975). It is the time when the individual learns to be autonomous, to be different from those close to her. Adolescence is most easily defined as the years between puberty and age 19 or between puberty and the achievement of intimacy (Erikson 1968). The onset of puberty is earlier now and thus the number of adolescents in our society is increasing. With puberty often comes sexual activity. It has been stated that 69% of 19-year-olds and 25% of 15-year-olds have had sexual intercourse (Flick 1986).

Adolescent Development

The girl who reaches puberty has many new tasks to master: to grow accustomed to her changing body and to the effects of hormonal rhythms and her monthly cycle; to recognize her fertility and the consequences of that fact; to acknowledge her responsibility; and to adjust to the different way others now view her. None of this is easy, especially in the years before her ability to reason abstractly develops.

Thus, for younger adolescents, action and its consequences and gratification and its delay are difficult concepts, often impossible to apply. Peer relationships are all-important at this time: She does not want to feel different or apart. She still tends to use fantasy and magical thinking, to hear facts and notice situations but to believe that she is different, somehow unique, and that nothing will happen to her that should not, especially pregnancy. By mid-adolescence she may be a dreamer, enjoying her new imaginative processes, idealizing her relationships and denying the need for contraception or rationalizing her biological susceptibility by wanting sex to be spontaneous and unplanned. Despite classes in sex education, she may use contraception improperly or become pregnant while using the birth-control pill and taking a medication that inhibits its effects. Some use no method of contraception, not only because of denial of the chance of pregnancy but because of a hope (conscious or unconscious) of becoming pregnant.

Franklin's (1988) extensive review of the literature revealed that adolescent females from families with low socioeconomic status and who were black were more often sexually active. Studies have also demonstrated that young, sexually active adolescents tended to do poorly in school, lived with large families or with one parent (usually the mother), drank and smoked early, came from lower-income families, and lived in large urban areas (Flick 1986; Zuckerman et al. 1984). In addition, they tended to prefer a nurturing role, wanted to please their male partner, and were looking for affection rather than sexual satisfaction. Their unhappiness at home led them to look for caring and identity through a relationship with a boyfriend. Most pregnancies were accidental, although sometimes the woman hoped the child would secure the relationship. Other authors have linked early pregnancy and poor school performance as indicators of hopelessness and the lack of belief in opportunities for employment (Group for the Advancement of Psychiatry 1986). Youngs (1980) noted that low self-esteem and poor academic achievement seemed to encourage pregnancy. A child provided a point from which the mother's life could be shaped: first child care, then maybe a job or job training, then adulthood.

Sally, at 21 the mother of a 4-year-old boy, said to her single-parent best friend, "When the children are teenagers and don't need to be babysat, then we can start dating men again. By then I will have a job and won't need to look for someone just to take care of me."

For others, parenthood means adulthood in the sense of feeling equal to their own mother or older sister. Employment, often difficult to obtain anyway, is now unnecessary. The majority of single mothers, however, do not want to rely on public assistance of any kind and, like Sally, wish to be further educated and employed. Many adolescents recognize the difficulties involved in raising children and request abortion. These young women sense their own immaturity and fear the psychological consequences of the months of pregnancy.

Adolescence is a time for developing a sense of self. The child must become accustomed to and comfortable with her changing body. She must absorb that these changes mean she is physically capable of becoming pregnant. She uses information from all sources, including parents, family, peers, the media, and schools. Thus she forms her own moral sense and eventually her own moral standards. This is all processed by and through her growing ability to reason and to use abstraction. The young adolescent is at a cognitive disadvantage, therefore, in her efforts to appreciate her physical development. She continues to believe that nothing unpleasant, such as pregnancy, could happen to her. Or she follows the examples set by older sisters or her mother and hopes to have a child.

Pregnancy

The youngster who lacks adequate self-esteem for any reason is very susceptible to peer pressure and unable to assert her own beliefs should she have formed some. She searches for affection and caring and gets a sense of value from taking care of another who seems to need her. This girl is likely to engage in sexual activity with a male who provides this opportunity for caring. As the adolescent searches for autonomy, she requires frequent reassurance that she is loved and valued. Many families cannot provide this because of their own internal problems, especially in many single-parent homes where the mother is struggling herself. The girl then seeks this caring elsewhere at a time when her sexuality is becoming more powerful and the means of attracting such loving attention. Thus when really wanting just to be cared about, to be held and to be able to cuddle, she becomes sexually involved through a sense of obligation or through force. Others equate caring with sexual expression or are unable to postpone sexual longings. Of course, this behavior is influenced by what they see around them and adopt as their own mode of behavior. Girls place a great deal of importance on relationships with others, and they look for involvements before young males are ready to do so. Gilligan (1982) outlined this need for intimacy clearly. This need is distinct from possessing an ability to share equally with another or to be able to deal with the vicissitudes of a relationship with another adult or an infant.

For the past 20 years, the number of unmarried adolescent girls who became pregnant has risen consistently. It has been estimated that if present trends continue, "40% of all 14 year olds in the United States would be pregnant at least once before they are 20" (Franklin 1988, p. 339). Interestingly, the rates for whites have increased, whereas those for blacks have decreased. Flick (1986) pointed out that even though a greater percentage of adolescent black women are sexually active and become pregnant more often, white adolescent women are increasingly becoming sexually active and thus more likely to become pregnant. Other authors have noted that sexual activity is beginning at an earlier age. Zuckerman et al. (1984) stated, "There has been a 22% increase in the birthrate for girls age 10–14 years, from 0.9 in 1966 to 1.1 in 1981" (p. 857). The birthrate for older adolescents decreased. Annually, 10% of all adolescent girls in the United States become pregnant. Put another way, "Each year more than 1 million adolescents age 15–19 in the United States become pregnant. Two-thirds of these pregnancies are conceived out of wedlock, and one-fifth of all births in the United States are to women still in their teens" (Group for the Advancement of Psychiatry 1986, p. 3).

This is a sizable proportion of young people. Despite the school classes in sexuality, the greater availability of contraceptive advice and devices, and the media dissemination of views and news of family planning, the impact on pregnancy rates has been minimal if at all. Obviously other, more influential, factors are at work here and must be examined.

The girl who becomes pregnant may so find herself for any of various reasons, and these will influence her subsequent decisions. As mentioned, the pregnancy may be a result of impulsivity not yet tempered by experience and the use of reasoning, a result of inattention to birth control by denying the personal possibility of pregnancy, or the desired result of a conscious decision to use pregnancy as an escape from home or to provide the girl with someone to love who will love her or make her an "adult" among her peers. In our technological society, sexual maturity does not necessarily coincide with psychological and social maturity (Miller and Simon 1980).

Decision Making

Once pregnant, the adolescent must decide to continue the pregnancy or have an abortion. If she decides the former, she will have to consider whether she wants to give the child up for adoption, but most adolescents today keep their babies. Many decide to have the pregnancy terminated. This decision is difficult for the girl who has not yet completed her individuation and is thus not accustomed to making autonomous choices. If living at home, she may be controlled by her parents' decisions, either to please them or because she requires their ongoing financial or emotional support. The adolescent who does not believe in abortion in theory may consider nothing but termination in reality, believing herself to be too young to tolerate a pregnancy. An older teenager will consider her options and may decide that the disruption pregnancy will mean in her present life is too great and then request an abortion. In some cases, the parents make the decision: abortion or adoption depending on their own beliefs, and sometimes the parents will consent to the infant living in their home. This is often socioculturally determined and influenced by the parents' needs as well.

The reason for becoming pregnant also influences the girl's decision. The youngster who acted impulsively or without thought to consequences may find herself facing the first serious decision of her life. Suddenly, she must deal with the results of her behavior. The girl who wanted someone to love her may rejoice in the prospect of a baby in this role, often with little idea of what motherhood entails. Similarly, the teenager who wishes to have a child because her sister or best friend does or for peer-group status to feel like an adult will view her pregnancy more positively.

Counseling

Proper counseling is, of course, necessary and ideal but not always available. When it is offered, the counselor must be aware of his or her own beliefs and consciously avoid allowing them to influence therapy. This may be difficult in a situation such as this one, which is so laden with emotions. Nevertheless, the adolescent is facing many pressures already, and the counseling session must offer her a safe place in which to explore her feelings freely.

All options must be explored: adoption, keeping the baby, and abortion. When possible, parental support should be sought and the family helped to deal with the event together. The adolescent should be encouraged to talk about her knowledge of and her fantasies of the fetus's development at that stage of pregnancy. She will discuss her ideas about the course of pregnancy and how she imagines she will feel. Such practical issues as where she can live during and after the pregnancy, whether she will remain in school or at a job, and how her friends and family will react must be brought forth. She will need to talk about the circumstances in which she became pregnant and about her feelings for the father of the fetus.

Discussions about the delivery and care of the newborn are important. The counselor should inquire about the girl's knowledge of infant behavior and needs. Constraints on her time and actions because of child care must be talked about, and so must financial needs. The girl's feelings about adoption as an option must also be explored.

The possibility of abortion as an option should be raised. The girl's previous beliefs about abortion and those of her family will need review and consideration. If she is considering abortion, the possible surgical procedures should be fully explained in a matter-of-fact manner. Any legal issues applicable in her home state must be outlined, as well as any need for parental consent. She may want to talk about her wish to inform the father of her pregnancy or about whether to involve him in her decision making.

The therapist's role is to enable the girl to explore and resolve any ambivalence she may have about the course and outcome of the pregnancy and to reach a decision with which she is comfortable. Thus involvement of the adolescent's parents may be important depending on the situation. Throughout the process, the therapist must remain acutely aware of his or her own feelings and counsel in a manner that is beneficial to the adolescent, regardless of the therapist's personal beliefs. Although this is a primary axiom in all psychotherapies, it is crucial in this situation.

In addition, the girl can be encouraged to talk about her sexuality, becoming pregnant, and future sexual behavior. Contraceptive advice and information should be given to her at this time. Finally, she must be told of the availability of therapy should she need it during the pregnancy and postpartum or after an abortion.

Outcome

Many youngsters keep their babies, but many younger girls (especially) decide on abortion. During the time when she is trying to make a decision, the girl will display features of depression, anxiety, and guilt as she weighs all of the issues involved. This can be very difficult for the immature adolescent (Group for the Advancement of Psychiatry 1986). She looks at her own beliefs about abortion; the importance she places on school, employment, socialization, and family relationships; and how she sees a pregnancy affecting all of this—as well as its effects on the rest of her life.

Afterward, having had the abortion, if she has been allowed to decide on an abortion without pressure from parents or others and has examined all of her options and feelings, she is usually relieved and experiences few emotional sequelae. Thus, despite early beliefs to the contrary, termination of pregnancy by abortion has not been shown to have long-lasting psychological effects, but it has shown symptoms of a brief, acute situational reaction (Greydanus and Railsback 1985; Group for the Advancement of Psychiatry 1986; Nadelson 1978; Poindexter and Kaufman 1980).

The adolescent who does do poorly after an abortion is the one who had been pushed by others (usually parents or a boyfriend) into a procedure that she did not want to have. The same statement could be made, however, about the girl who carries a baby for the full term against her wishes: She experiences regret, sorrow, guilt, and anger.

Teenage pregnancy is not without risk. Teenagers have many more complications during pregnancy than do adult women because of their physical immaturity and poor health habits. Risks to the adolescent mother and her child are dependent on socioeconomic factors, nutritional habits, and substance and alcohol abuse; all of these areas carry greater risks in that age group in any case. The younger adolescent especially has a greater chance of giving birth to a premature small baby with neonatal complications (Martin and Valente 1987; Miller and Field 1985; Zuckerman et al. 1984).

This greater chance is closely related to poor health habits and emphasizes the need for adequate prenatal counseling. Studies have shown, however, that teenagers have lower rates of morbidity and mortality from the procedures for inducing abortion than do older women. This is true even when gestational age is adjusted for; adolescents characteristically have later abortions because of their initial denial or unawareness of the pregnancy (Cates et al. 1983).

Prevention

Flick (1986) stated that "an abortion is now elected in 38% of all adolescent pregnancies. . . . Only 49% of adolescent pregnancies lead to live birth; the remaining 14% end in miscarriage or stillbirth" (p. 133). More younger than older adolescents choose abortion, and the older ones usually keep their child to raise themselves. Girls who are doing well in school and see a future for themselves occupationally and educationally are more often those who chose abortion (Flick 1986; Nadelson et al. 1978). In these adolescents, the choice of abortion is a decision allowing movement toward autonomy and individuation, an expression of self-esteem and confidence in their own future.

The adolescent who chooses to raise her own child must be provided with counseling about physical and psychological health factors for herself and her child. She must also be guided toward continued schooling and future employment to alleviate some of the socioeconomic factors that may have led to the pregnancy.

Present health education is schools is inadequate, given the number of teenage pregnancies. More advice about contraception needs to be spread through acceptable channels for adolescents, such as television, videotapes, and other media. Furthermore, contraceptive methods need to be available to these youngsters easily. They are sexually active, as the statistics reveal. Denying them easy access to contraception only increases the pregnancy rate. Above all, health care professionals should be constantly aware of the adolescent's sexuality and use any consultation opportunity to open a discussion of sexual activity and feelings. Knowledge of the factors placing an adolescent at high risk immediately heightens the health care professional's ability to spot and counsel the youngster. Primary prevention is the most important goal—alleviation of the psychological and socioeconomic factors that are such strong determinants of adolescent sexual activity. That demands political, not just educational, change. In the end, we must offer teenagers the benefit of our knowledge, reasoned unbiased counsel, and, when necessary, therapy suitable to their developmental status.

References

Cates W, Schulz KF, Grimes DA: The risk associated with teenage abortion. N Engl J Med 309:621–624, 1983

Erikson E: Identity: Youth and Crisis. New York, WW Norton, 1968

Flick LH: Paths to adolescent parenthood: implications for prevention. Public Health Rep 101:132–147, 1986

Franklin DL: Race, class and adolescent pregnancy: an ecological analysis. Am J Orthopsychiatry 58:339–354, 1988

Gilligan C: In a Different Voice. Cambridge, MA, Harvard University Press, 1982

Greydanus DE, Railsback LD: Abortion in adolescence. Seminars in Adolescent Medicine 1:213–222, 1985

Group for the Advancement of Psychiatry: Crisis of adolescence: teenage pregnancy: impact on adolescent development (Report 118). New York, Brunner/Mazel, 1986

Martin LS, Valente CM: "Life-style" and pregnancy outcome in adolescents. Maryland Med J 36:943–950, 1987

Miller KA, Field CS: Adolescent pregnancy: critical review for the clinician. Seminars in Adolescent Medicine 1:195–212, 1985

Miller PY, Simon W: The development of sexuality in adolescence, in Handbook of Adolescent Psychology. Edited by Adelson J. New York, John Wiley, 1980, pp 383–407

Nadelson CC: The emotional impact of abortion, in the Woman Patient: Medical and Psychological Interfaces, Vol 1. Edited by Notman MT, Nadelson CC. New York, Plenum, 1978, pp 173–179

Nadelson CC, Notman MT, Gillon J: Adolescent sexuality and pregnancy, in The Woman Patient: Medical and Psychological Interfaces, Vol 1. Edited by Notman MT, Nadelson CC. New York, Plenum, 1978, pp 123–130

Offer D, Offer JB: From Teenage to Young Manhood: A Psychological Study. New York, Basic Books, 1975

Poindexter AN, Kaufman RH: Issues surrounding adolescent pregnancy termination, in Adolescent Pregnancy: Perspectives for the Health Professional. Edited by Smith PB, Mumford DM. Boston, MA, GK Hall, 1980

Youngs DD: Psychiatric aspects of adolescent pregnancy, in Adolescent Pregnancy: Perspectives for the Health Professional. Edited by Smith PB, Mumford DM. Boston, MA, GK Hall, 1980

Zuckerman BS, Walker DK, Frank DA, et al: Adolescent pregnancy: biobehavioral determinants of outcome. J Pediatr 105:857–863, 1984

Chapter 14

Abortion: Ethical Issues for Clinicians

John D. Lantos, M.D.
Christine L. McHenry, M.D.
Carl Elliott, M.D.

Dora Klein is a 22-year-old single female who has asked to see a psychiatrist during an obstetric clinic visit in which she learned that she is 13 weeks pregnant. An ultrasound reading during her clinic visit has revealed the possibility of neural tube anomalies.

Clearly agitated and anxious about her pregnancy, she makes a comment during the interview about cutting her wrists, but when she is questioned she denies any suicidal plans. She has been living with a man for 2 months, but she says that she does not know who the father of the child is.

Records from a previous psychiatric hospitalization indicate a possible diagnosis of borderline personality disorder. She complains of long-standing feelings of emptiness and boredom, and she has had several brief periods of depression that lasted only a few days. She has seen several psychiatrists and claims that she stopped seeing the last one after he made sexual advances toward her.

Married and divorced twice, she has lived with various other men during the past 2 years, the longest relationship lasting 3 months. Her history is also significant for substance abuse and for self-mutilation during periods of stress.

Moral analysis of the abortion debate is often framed in terms of absolute moral principles, such as the sanctity of life, the personhood of the fetus, or the autonomy of the mother. By framing the discussion in these terms, ethical dilemmas become conflicts between irreconcilable principles, such as the fetus's right to life and the mother's right to choose. Real ethical dilemmas do not arise in the abstract, however. Instead, they arise in the complex lives of real people living in unique communities at particular historical moments. Attempts to separate ethics and morality from the rest of life, and to speak of disembodied and contextless moral principles, ignore the complexities of moral decision making. Rather than resolving ethical dilemmas, they lead to endless and fruitless debate, such as we have seen over abortion in recent years.

There is an alternative approach to moral philosophy that, while not ignoring ethical principles and norms, seeks understanding of moral problems by analysis of the particular context in which they arise. By this approach, when a person is faced with moral problems, his or her life history, interrelationships with moral communities, and personal values are as pertinent as the principles of philosophers in arriving at a sensible and morally defensible decision. This approach requires a practical moral reasoning process similar to the practical medical reasoning required of physicians who assess patients and arrive at medically defensible decisions. Before describing how this process should work, it is necessary to dispel a few possible misconceptions about what such a clinical ethics process is and is not.

Clinical Ethics Is Not Risk-Benefit Assessment

To start, good ethical analysis must begin with facts about the natural history of disease and about the risks and benefits of proposed treatments. Such data will allow physicians to calculate the indications or contraindications for abortion given particular case presentations—in the context of maternal acquired immunodeficiency syndrome (AIDS), diabetes, multiple gestations, and severe maternal depression. Such calculations must be the starting point of any clinical decision making. In many situations, there are no precise data on the implications of decisions to continue or terminate a pregnancy. For example, the risk of infection in the baby of a mother who is seropositive for the human immunodeficiency virus varies widely. Similarly, the prognosis for a woman who appears suicidal over a recently diagnosed pregnancy will be, at best, an estimate of the likelihood of one outcome over another, not a definite prediction that one outcome will occur. As in all clinical decisions, the range of uncertainty must be considered in deciding how data should be interpreted to make the best recommendation for a particular patient.

Risk-benefit data will influence clinical decisions but cannot, by themselves, determine whether a procedure is morally acceptable. Moral reasoning must go much further; it might include explicit consideration of the patient's values, the goals of therapy, social or economic factors, and possibly societal values.

Clinical Ethics Is Not a Public Opinion Poll

It is also important to distinguish clinical ethics from social science data about the beliefs and attitudes of various segments of the population about abortion. Although moral values should, in general, reflect community values, there are two important reasons why moral analysis requires more than a public opinion poll. First, moral analysis should not merely describe what people do or think. It should show what people ought to do and think. Second, although good moral analysis should lead to rules for what most people ought to do in most situations, it must also guide individuals in particular situations. Thus, the moral proscription against killing might be interpreted differently for soldiers, policemen, or judges than for others.

Like risk-benefit data and prognostic assessments, social science data may help us frame moral arguments. Where community consensus is broad, there may be a higher burden of proof on the individual who disagrees with the community values to justify his or her beliefs through moral reasoning. Where consensus does not exist, as in the abortion debate, the burden of moral argument lies more with those who would impose their values on others. In both situations, attitude surveys may set constraints on but do not replace or predetermine moral reasoning.

Clinical Ethics Is Not Relativism

The case-based approach has established itself in medicine without leading to therapeutic relativism; however, some see any deviation from moral rules as a sign of moral relativism. For centuries, tension has existed between those who would apply moral principles absolutely and those who were sensitive to the extenuating circumstances of life stories. Martha Nussbaum, a contemporary classicist, describes the disagreement between Plato and Aristotle over this issue. "Plato . . . is committed to the idea that what is *truly* and intrinsically valuable is so always and from a perspective totally severed from particular context," Nussbaum wrote, whereas for Aristotle, "The things that are good and valuable may not be so relatively to all imaginable ways and conditions of life. The good of some genuine values may be context-relative and not any the less good for that" (Nussbaum 1986, p. 293).

The difference between these philosophers may be best illustrated by their attitudes toward tragic drama. In Plato's ideal republic, playwrights would be banished; for Aristotle, the tragedies represent a refined moral wisdom. Aristotle's respect for tragedy illustrates his belief that moral dilemmas are best understood by careful examination of complex situations in which profound moral values are in conflict and where our choices may be limited to actions that all seem profoundly wrong.

In a perfect world, nobody would ever want or need an abortion. As anthropologist Clifford Geertz wrote, "Those of us who are opposed to increased legal restrictions on abortion are not, I take it, pro-abortion, in the sense that we think abortion a wonderful thing and hold that the greater the abortion rate, the greater the well-being of society" (Geertz 1984, p. 263). To be, in Geertz's words, "anti-anti-abortion" is to acknowledge the need for elasticity and for occasionally making choices in situations where every choice seems wrong. In such situations, the tragedy arises precisely because every choice is wrong, yet we must choose. An analogy can be made to other moral dilemmas. For example, Leszak Kolakowski, a political scientist, acknowledges that "lying is evil and sometimes it is better to lie, knowing that lying is evil, in order to prevent an even greater evil, and in those circumstances, lying, whether morally permissible or not, never ceases to be evil" (Kolakowski 1973, p. 221).

Twentieth-century revisionist theologians have grappled with the distinction between a desire to adhere to moral principles and the need for sensitivity to the uniqueness of life stories. They argue for a distinction between moral evil and premoral evil (Gula 1988). For example, killing is an act of premoral evil. It has the potential of being evil, but it can only be judged so by looking at the circumstances of the act. If someone kills out of jealousy, our moral evaluation of the act will be different from what it would be if that person killed in self-defense. In the latter case, we see that the act of killing represents a choice between two abhorrent acts—taking another's life or meaninglessly sacrificing one's own. In the former situation, no such proportion of disvalue versus value exists. By this approach, moral norms ("Do not kill") continue to illuminate how one ought to act, but the uniqueness of the circumstances and the intent of the actor will determine if the act is justifiable.

The case-based approach to moral decisions is not in conflict with but is complementary to principle-based approaches to ethics. Because any threat to the legalistic or principle-based approaches raises the specter of relativism—that is, the threat of a world in which there is no concept of the right and the good beyond personal preferences—many people find the case-based approach threatening. Geertz (1984) summed up this fear as the belief that "if something isn't anchored everywhere then nothing can be anchored anywhere" (p. 265). Instead, case-based ethics should be seen as the practical moral reasoning necessary when moral principles are in conflict and action is necessary.

Clinical Ethics and Clinical Science

In a way, this approach to ethics is more modest than the daring and comprehensive systems of theoretical philosophers. It plods along, much as clinical science plods along. Its principles and maxims emerge from observation of life stories. Just as, by observation of health and disease, we learn the signs and symptoms of pathology and the habits that lead to health, so, from observation of exemplary behavior, we begin to discern the rules that seem to allow people to live good and virtuous lives in harmony with one another. Eventually, after refinement by scientists, theologians, philosophers, and common sense, life stories become refined into maxims, parables, principles, and cases that come to serve a prescriptive function, telling us how we ought to live in order to achieve health or virtue. For physicians, who know that the world is a messy and surprising place, questions should arise about the presumption that comprehensive moral codes are possible.

In an insightful review of the development of moral philosophy, Alasidair MacIntyre (1984) showed that attempts to derive comprehensive moral systems are a relatively recent phenomenon of moral philosophy. He discussed a precursor of such moral systems, the ancient Greek concept of virtue. Virtue, according to MacIntyre, can only be defined in relation to particular practices—there is no free-floating virtue and no abstract or disembodied notion of the good. "The exercise of a virtue exhibits qualities which are required for sustaining a social role: to excel is to excel at war or in the games, as Achilles does, in sustaining a household, as Penelope does, in giving counsel in the assembly, as Nestor does, in the telling of a tale, as Homer himself does" (MacIntyre 1984, p. 187).

Physicians should easily grasp the conceptual basis for such a moral system. Many of our most difficult moral conflicts arise out of the particular obligations we take on as physicians. One of these obligations is to respect our patients' values in order to do what is best for the patient. Dilemmas arise, however, when a patient's values or ideas of what is best conflict with our own. In the course of our work, conflicts may arise, for example, between our obligations to tell the truth and our wish to protect a patient from knowledge that may be painful, or between our obligations to relieve pain and to preserve life.

Stephen Toulmin, a philosopher and historian of science, argued that, by "reintroducing into ethical debate the vexed topics raised by *particular cases*, [bioethics] obliged philosophers to address once again the Aristotelian problems of *practical reasoning*, which had been on the sidelines for too long" (Toulmin 1982, p. 749). By doing so, Toulmin stated, medicine "saved the life of ethics" (p. 750).

In a more recent book, Toulmin collaborated with Al Jonsen, a theologian and medical ethicist, to develop further the analogy between thought processes necessary for case-based moral philosophy and the thought processes of clinical medicine (Jonsen and Toulmin 1988). They make clear that, just because physicians arrive at different diagnoses and therapeutic plans for different patients, they are not practicing relativistic medicine.

Instead, physicians constantly move, intellectually, among the scientific theory, medical facts, professional values, and the particularities of the case as they decide on a diagnosis and a plan of treatment. Facts and theories constrain the possible responses to a clinical dilemma, but personal and professional values finally determine the outcome of the doctor-patient encounter.

The Physician's Role in Abortion Decisions

Few moral analyses of abortion focus on the physician's moral choice to perform or not to perform an abortion. This is curious, because the necessity of the physician's participation is a crucial aspect of the debate. If a woman could induce an abortion alone in her room without any physician participation, the moral calculus of abortion debates would change. Moral considerations derived from the physician-patient relationship, such as the need for trust and mutual respect, would simply vanish. Furthermore, the entire regulatory structure, by which legal sanctions against abortion are directed at physicians, not patients, would become obsolete.

In the wake of the U.S. Supreme Court *Webster v. Reproductive Health Services* (1989) decision, it is likely that state regulation of abortion will allow for greater physician control over abortion decisions. As a result, many physicians will soon be confronted with cases in which they will be able, through a medical opinion, either to sanction or to prohibit an abortion. Individual doctors will be called on in different capacities. The obstetrician and the perinatologist may be called on to assess fetal viability. The geneticist may need to describe the anticipated health problems of a fetus with chromosomal anomalies. The psychiatrist may be asked to determine whether continuing a pregnancy will jeopardize a woman's mental health. Physicians will participate in different types of cases—for example, unplanned pregnancy, genetically defective fetuses, maternal AIDS, or severe maternal depression. Each type of case will raise particular medical and moral issues.

The physician's participation in abortion decisions locates those decisions within the moral domain of the doctor-patient relationship. Within this domain, ethical questions arise from the unique duties and obligations of doctors to their patients. The conflicts that arise reflect a clash between important and often irreconcilable values. On the one hand, physicians have obligations to act in such a way as to maximize their patients' well-being and to respect their patients' autonomy. These obligations are implicit and central to the sharing, trusting, and beneficent doctor-patient relationship. On the other hand, physicians may feel bound by religious beliefs, professional oaths, or moral obligations to preserve fetal life that conflict with their judgment about what is best for the patient.

For physicians, then, practical ethical reasoning is the stuff of daily life, and the ethical issues in abortion decisions are best approached as we approach other clinical ethical issues. We must carefully consider the medical data about the indications and contraindications for abortion, from physiologic and psychiatric perspectives. We must elicit and interpret the patient's preferences and try to understand the life circumstances that led to the tragic decision to terminate a pregnancy. We must examine our own moral values. Finally, we must go beyond reflection and introspection and act.

Many of our actions have effects that are irreversible. In this, perhaps, lies the most compelling justification for a moral sensitivity rooted not in our principles but in the patient's life story. We must live with our recommendations only theoretically or in memory, but for the patient, the clinical decision will shape her life. A William Carlos Williams poem illustrates the moral complexity of such decisions and the paradoxical simplicity that may result when we settle on a diagnosis and a plan (Williams 1984):

A Cold Front

This woman with a dead face
has seven foster children
and a new baby of her own in
spite of that. She wants pills

for an abortion and says,
Um Hum, in reply to me while
her blanketed infant makes
unrelated grunts of salutation.

She looks at me with her mouth
open and blinks her expressionless
carved eyes, like a cat
on a limb too tired to go higher

from its tormentors. And still
the baby chortles in its spit
and there is a dull flush
almost of beauty to the woman's face

as she says, looking at me
quietly, I won't have any more.
In a case like this I know
quick action is the main thing.

References

Geertz CL: Anti-anti relativism. American Anthropologist 86:263–278, 1984
Gula R: What Are They Saying About Moral Norms? New York, Paulist Press, 1988, pp 61–81

Jonsen A, Toulmin S: The Abuse of Casuistry. Berkeley, CA, University of California Press, 1988

Kolakowski L: Ethics without a moral code. Triquarterly 43:221, 1973

MacIntyre A: After Virtue: A Study in Moral Theory, 2nd Edition. South Bend, IN, University of Notre Dame Press, 1984

Nussbaum MC: The Fragility of Goodness: Luck and Ethics in Greek Tragedy and Philosophy. Cambridge, UK, Cambridge University Press, 1986

Toulmin S: How medicine saved the life of ethics. Perspect Biol Med 25:736–750, 1982

Webster v. Reproductive Health Services, 109 S.Ct. 3040 (1989)

Williams WC: The Doctor Stories. Edited by Coles R. New York, New Directions, 1984, p 131

Index